# The Natural Estrogen Diet

## Ordering

Trade bookstores in the U.S. and Canada, please contact:

Publishers Group West
1700 Fourth Street, Berkeley, CA 94710
Phone: (800) 788-3123
Fax: (510) 528-3444

Hunter House books are available at bulk discounts for textbook course adoption; to qualifying community, healthcare, and government organizations; and for special promotions and fundraising. For details, please contact:

Special Sales Department
Hunter House Inc.
P. O. Box 2914, Alameda, CA 94501-0914
Phone: (510) 865-5282
Fax: (510) 865-4295
e-mail: marketing@hunterhouse.com

Individuals can order our books from most bookstores or by calling toll free:
(800) 266-5592

# The Natural Estrogen Diet

### Healthy Recipes for Perimenopause and Menopause

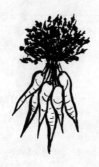

## DR. LANA LIEW
### with LINDA OJEDA, PH.D.

Hunter House PUBLISHERS

**Library of Congress Cataloging-in-Publication Data**
Liew, Lana
    The natural estrogen diet : healthy recipes for perimenopause and menopause /
Lana Liew with Linda Ojeda. — 1st ed.
        p. cm.
    Rev. ed. of : The natural estrogen book / Lana Liew. East Roseville, N.S.W. :
Simon & Schuster, 1998.
    Includes bibliographical references and index.
    ISBN 0-89793-246-3
    1. Menopause—Complications—Diet therapy—Recipes. 2. Perimenopause—
Complications—Diet therapy—Recipes. 3. Menopause—Complications—
Alternative treatment. 4. Menopause—Hormone therapy. 5.
Menopause—Nutritional aspects. 6. Estrogen—Therapeutic use. 7. Middle aged
women—Health and hygiene.
    I. Ojeda, Linda. II. Liew, Lana. Natural estrogen book. III. Title.
RG186.L465 1999
618.1'750654—dc 21                                              98-52737
                                                                CIP

*Cover Design:* Jil Weil Designs, Oakland      *Book Production:* Terragraphics
*Editor:* Laura Harger                         *Recipe Editor:* Naomi Wise
*Proofreader:* Lee Rappold                     *Indexer:* Kathy Talley-Jones
*Managing Editor:* Wendy Low                   *Editorial Assistant:* Jennifer Rader
*Acquisitions Coordinator:* Jeanne Brondino    *Nutrient Analysis:* Amy Demmon
*Publicity Director:* Marisa Spatafore         *Marketing Intern:* Monique Portegies
*Customer Support:* Christina Sverdrup, Joel Irons
*Order Fulfillment:* A & A Quality Shipping Services
*Publisher:* Kiran S. Rana

Printed and Bound by: Publishers Press, Salt Lake City, Utah
Manufactured in the United States of America

9 8 7 6 5 4 3 2 1     First U.S. Edition     99 00 01 02 03

# Contents

Acknowledgments . . . . . . . . . . . . . . . . . . . . . . . . . . . . . . . .   vii

Foreword . . . . . . . . . . . . . . . . . . . . . . . . . . . . . . . . . . . . . . .   ix

Introduction . . . . . . . . . . . . . . . . . . . . . . . . . . . . . . . . . . .   1

PART I—NATURAL ESTROGENS . . . . . . . . . . . . . . .   7

Chapter One—Estrogen Foods and Menopause . . . . . . .   9

Chapter Two—Plant Hormones and Other Health
Concerns for Women . . . . . . . . . . . . . . . . . . . . . . . . . . . . .   25

Chapter Three—An Introduction to Soy . . . . . . . . . . . .   43

Chapter Four—Integrating Natural Estrogens Into
Your Life . . . . . . . . . . . . . . . . . . . . . . . . . . . . . . . . . . . . . .   53

PART II—RECIPES . . . . . . . . . . . . . . . . . . . . . . . . . . .   65

    Glossary of Ingredients . . . . . . . . . . . . . . . . . . . . . . .   69

    Basic Recipes . . . . . . . . . . . . . . . . . . . . . . . . . . . . . . . .   75

    Appetizers, Snacks, and Pick-Me-Ups . . . . . . . . . . . .   81

    Soups . . . . . . . . . . . . . . . . . . . . . . . . . . . . . . . . . . . . . .   93

    Salads, Dressings, and Side Dishes . . . . . . . . . . . . . .   103

    Main Courses . . . . . . . . . . . . . . . . . . . . . . . . . . . . . . .   129

    Pancakes, Breads, and Muffins . . . . . . . . . . . . . . . . .   175

    Desserts . . . . . . . . . . . . . . . . . . . . . . . . . . . . . . . . . . . .   187

Health Glossary . . . . . . . . . . . . . . . . . . . . . . . . . . . . . . . .   198

Resources . . . . . . . . . . . . . . . . . . . . . . . . . . . . . . . . . . . . . .   202

References . . . . . . . . . . . . . . . . . . . . . . . . . . . . . . . . . . . . . .   204

Appendix: A simplified diagram showing the
    phytoestrogens that are currently known to
    be important to humans . . . . . . . . . . . . . . . . . . . . . .   208

Index . . . . . . . . . . . . . . . . . . . . . . . . . . . . . . . . . . . . . . . . . .   209

# Important Notice

The material in this book is intended to provide information regarding nutrition and diet. Every effort has been made to provide accurate and dependable information. The contents of this book have been compiled using professional research and in consultation with medical professionals. However, healthcare professionals have differing opinions and advances in medical and scientific research are made very quickly, so some of the information may become outdated.

Therefore, the publisher, authors, editors, and professionals quoted in the book cannot be held responsible for any error, omission, or dated material. The authors and publisher assume no responsibility for any outcome of applying the information in this book in a program of self-care or under the care of a licensed practitioner. If you have questions concerning your nutrition or diet, or about the application of the information described in this book, consult a qualified healthcare professional.

# Acknowledgments

Many scientists throughout the world have worked tirelessly in the research of phytoestrogen-containing foods and their effects on the health of men and women. They are too numerous to name, but each and every one of them has contributed to the knowledge from which this book draws—the research into disease prevention using pure extracts of isoflavones and other plant products.

My eldest daughter, Camilla, was most enthusiastic about this book and she spurred me on with it. Her encouragement and support are most appreciated, not to mention her help with research, proofreading and tasting of the recipes.

I would also like to thank my two younger daughters, who understood that their time with their mother had to be shared with a compelling project. They, too, have been most patient and supportive.

Special thanks are due to the following friends: Margaret, Bev, Nanny, Annie, Siew Fong, Stephanie and Christopher, who have shared their recipes, thoughts and interest. Above all, their belief and support have been vital in the development of this book. Many patients have also encouraged me along the way.

Acknowledgments of help are also due to the following: Dora Spilbergs for proofreading and useful comments; Evan Black for help with some research articles; Grahame and Lyndall Black for sustaining encouragement and interest; Jenny Chan, Consultant Dietitian-Nutritionist (B.Sc., Masters in Nutrition and Dietetics, MDAA, APD), for her work and contribution to the analysis of the recipes; Dr. Randall Fray for his interest and enthusiasm in the book; Professor John Eden for his helpful suggestions and comments; and David Rosenberg, Brigitta Doyle and Siobhan O'Connor at Simon & Schuster for their assistance in the production of the Australian edition of this book.

— Lana Liew

I would like to acknowledge the many contributors who supplied recipes for our collection: the Ohio Soybean Council, the Indiana Soybean Board, Vitasoy, Azumaya, Dana Jacobi, and Laura Nilsen. A special tribute goes to Naomi Wise, for supplying a few of her own recipes and for her expert advice, and to both Naomi and Laura Harger for the Americanization of the original text. I would also like to thank the staff at Hunter House and express particular gratitude to Wendy Low and Amy Demmon, for their painstaking efforts and patience in working with the nutritional analysis software program. And, finally, to my publisher, Kiran Rana. We did it again—another wonderful collaborative effort.

— *Linda Ojeda*

# Foreword

The latest focus in nutrition research is on phytoestrogens. Phytoestrogens are a diverse group of plant-derived substances that have estrogenic activity in animals. These compounds are similar to estrogens and are characterized by their ability to elicit a specific response in estrogen-sensitive tissues. There is a great deal of interest in the potential benefits of dietary phytoestrogens in hormone-dependent processes. Animals have been known to graze selectively on plants to enhance or diminish fertility. Much of the early research on phytoestrogens was done with animals and interest was induced by the observation that sheep who grazed too much on clover became infertile. Epidemiological studies have shown that the incidence of hormone-dependent diseases is significantly lower in Asian populations whose diets are high in phytoestrogen consumption. Further studies comparing native Asian women to other cultures have suggested that the high phytoestrogen content of their diets may be responsible in part for their low rate of breast cancer and the ease with which they pass through menopause.

Phytoestrogens have both weak estrogenic and anti-estrogenic activity. Estradiol, our bodies' strongest estrogen, can be released from the ovary and travel to any number of target tissues, including the breast and uterus. At the breast, the estradiol can bind to the receptor site and increase cell division; at the uterus, estradiol can cause the endometrial lining to thicken. However, not all substances have a positive effect on the target tissue. Such is the case with Tamoxifen, a drug which is used in the treatment of breast cancer. Tamoxifen can bind to the estrogen receptors of the breast without causing any increase in cell division, thereby acting as an "estrogen blocker." At the same time, it can bind to receptors in the uterus and cause proliferation of the endometrium. Tamoxifen therefore has an antiestrogenic effect on the breast, but a proestrogenic effect on the uterus.

The most commonly studied phytoestrogens include the isoflavonoids, lignans, and coumestans found in high amounts in soybeans, flaxseed, and alfalfa, and also in many other vegetables and fruits. Much of the original research was targeted at menopausal women. Phytoestrogens have an estrogenic effect on the vaginal epithelium similar to that seen in patients treated with hormone replacement therapy. There is evidence, too, that hot flashes are resolved. Phytoestrogens also exert a cardiovascular protective effect by regulating lipid levels. Dietary soy supplementation has been shown to increase bone mineral density. Phytoestrogens may also protect against some types of cancer. Finally, there is evidence that there is a lower incidence of breast, colon, and prostate cancer in Asia, where soy intake is high in comparison to Western countries, where intake is relatively low.

Certainly, more studies of women using phytoestrogens need to be done to establish both the benefits and risks. However, given the bulk of information available, the use of phytoestrogens in a well-balanced diet may be considered a relatively safe method of effecting estrogen activity.

— *Dr. Randall E. Fray, M.B., Ch.B.,*
*F.R.C.O.G., F.R.A.C.O.G.*
*Gynecologist*
*Bankstown, Australia*

# Introduction

Hormone replacement therapy (HRT) is a popular discussion topic among women, particularly those who are menopausal or peri-menopausal (in the years immediately before the onset of meno-pause). HRT, which is taken in order to reduce some of the bothersome symptoms associated with menopause—hot flashes, mood swings, and the like—attempts to compensate for the falling level of estrogen production that accompanies menopause, but it is not suitable for every woman. To take HRT or not to take it? That is the driving question.

Some women are quite content with their HRT program, and they should continue with the regimen, under their doctor's supervision. However, some women have tried HRT in various combinations and forms and to their disappointment have been forced to stop because of numerous undesirable side effects. There are also those for whom HRT is definitely forbidden (women with certain kinds of cancer, for example), and thus they don't have this option. And finally, a growing number of women view meno-pause as a natural transition that does not require outside hor-monal intervention. This book is designed to help those women who cannot tolerate hormones, cannot take hormones, or simply choose not to medicate, yet who are concerned about controlling menopausal symptoms, preserving bone integrity, and preventing heart disease. Alternatives to HRT—using natural foods and lifestyle changes—can address all of these concerns, and this book describes some of these options.

Widespread interest in nonmedical treatments for an ever-growing number of conditions is sweeping the country. Pre-menopausal women who have no other option than to utilize alternative methods are clamoring for specific information and guidance. Many have read magazine articles that speak about foods that can potentially alter estrogen levels in the body, but details are scant. Which foods elicit what response, women ask, and how much of a particular food must be eaten to be effective? This book answers both these questions, based on the latest available scientific information.

*The Natural Estrogen Diet* discusses a variety of foods that are rich in naturally occurring plant estrogens (known as phytoestrogens). It explains how these gentle estrogenlike substances can work to minimize menopausal symptoms while also benefiting the bones and the heart and possibly curbing the risk of breast cancer. Of course, nutritional information is useless unless you have a practical plan for implementing changes in your daily diet, so this book also provides a number of suggestions—from the simplest, quickest, and easiest dietary changes to more involved and creative recipes—for altering your eating habits.

The first step in the natural estrogen diet is to look at the list on page 17 of foods that contain these health-promoting substances. Consider how many of these foods are already part of your regular diet, and determine ways to integrate some of the other foods into your daily meals and snacks.

The second step is to learn about soy products. Research has found that soy contains the most potent isoflavones, a subclass of plant estrogens that are thought to be responsible for many health benefits. For this reason, this book focuses on easy and tasty ways to add soy to your life. Soy may be foreign to your palate now, but we hope that you will remain open-minded and try something new and exciting, especially since soy has the potential for aiding your health in so many ways. Consider some of the possible benefits of soy:

❖ Soy has been shown to reduce hot flashes and other menopausal symptoms in some women.

❖ Soy has been shown to reduce coronary heart disease rates and lower high blood pressure and elevated cholesterol in human subjects.

❖ Soy increases bone density in postmenopausal women and may protect them from osteoporosis.

❖ Animal studies suggest that soy works as well as HRT to keep arteries to the brain free of cholesterol; thus, it may prevent stroke.

❖ Soy may help to fight breast cancer. Rates of breast cancer are lower in Asia and other regions where soy foods are eaten in large quantities.

❖ Soy may be instrumental in preventing other cancers, such as endometrial cancer in women, prostate cancer in men, and colon cancer.

## What Are the Advantages of the Natural Estrogen Diet?

❖ It is completely natural, and you can use the diet without fear of contraindications or the side effects that you may experience with HRT.

❖ The foods are readily available and do not require prescriptions or a visit to a health practitioner.

❖ Phytoestrogens are present in a wide variety of healthy foods, which also contain other beneficial compounds such as natural vitamins, minerals, antioxidants, healthy fats, and fiber.

❖ Some of the foods in the diet contain plant progestins as well. Examples are red clover, thyme, and turmeric. Progestins are hormones that behave like progesterone. Progesterone is the other hormone produced by women in significant amounts during the second half of the menstrual cycle, and its levels also fall during perimenopause and menopause.

❖ The natural estrogen diet is less costly than HRT.

❖   The diet has psychological as well as physical benefits. You are
    helping yourself without taking medications or drugs in order
    to feel "normal."

## What Are the Disadvantages of the
## Natural Estrogen Diet?

❖   Doses are not standardized in natural or manufactured foods.
    Researchers are still exploring the amount of phytoestrogen
    that is sufficient to produce health benefits. Conventional
    HRT tablets and patches, on the other hand, do come in stan-
    dard doses which also require titration in many users.

❖   Changing eating habits is inconvenient for some women, who
    may rely on swallowing a tablet or slapping on a patch to rem-
    edy their symptoms. This could be due to an attitudinal prob-
    lem or simply a lack of time.

❖   Certain foods or ingredients in the diet may be difficult to
    obtain or prepare.

❖   There is a general lack of knowledge about how to prepare and
    use the diet's foods and ingredients.

❖   Effectiveness may vary, depending upon the plant products
    used and also upon individual factors. Absorption of phytoe-
    strogens, for example, depends on the amount of time food
    takes to pass through the intestines, the status of the gut, the
    presence of appropriate bacteria in the intestines, and the
    amount of chemicals in the plant product, which is influenced
    by the plant's genetic origin and the climactic and environ-
    mental conditions under which it grew.

❖   It takes a few months before individuals start to experience
    the benefits of the natural estrogen diet. The diet is not as fast-
    acting as HRT, and people often find it difficult to wait for
    results.

❖ Some individuals may experience flatulence (gas) during the early days of the diet if they start the diet too quickly or eat overly large portions of the foods.

Chapter One, Menopause and Estrogen Foods, discusses some of the symptoms that can accompany menopause and explains how phytoestrogens—particularly those found in soy foods—work to alleviate menopause-related problems. Chapter Two, Plant Hormones and Other Health Concerns for Women, discusses these substances' other promising benefits—they can help protect against heart disease, osteoporosis, and even cancer. Chapter Three introduces you to soy foods, and Chapter Four guides you through easy ways to integrate them into your daily diet (here, too, you'll find detailed nutritional information on soy products). Finally, Part Two provides a wide range of recipes that will help you make soy and other phytoestrogen-containing foods a permanent—and delicious—part of your life.

We wish you good luck with your new dietary plan and your experimental tasting and cooking, and we also wish you many years of good health, delight, and enjoyment of the natural estrogen diet.

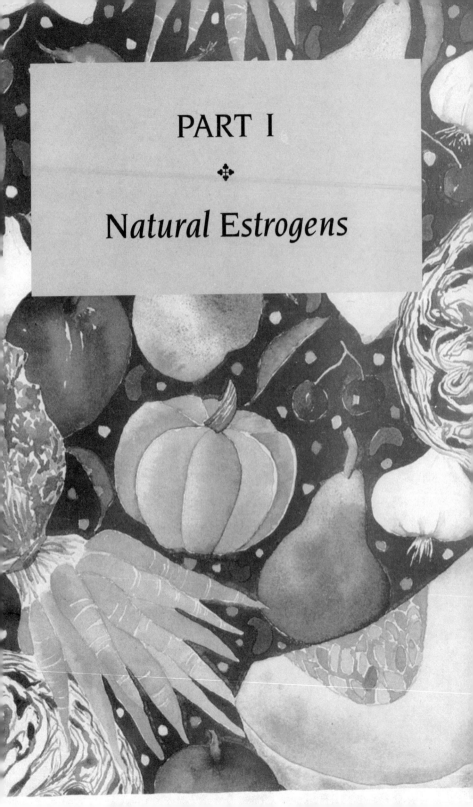

# PART I

✤

# Natural Estrogens

# CHAPTER ONE

## Estrogen Foods
## and Menopause

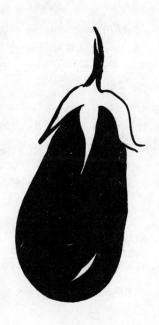

## Symptoms of Menopause

Some women remember hearing about menopause from their mothers, aunts, or older friends. Others may have read about the general physical process and seen personal stories in women's magazines and newspapers or heard them on the radio or television. A smaller contingent may have even attended a full-day seminar or weekend retreat on the topic, where women shared their own personal journeys and discussed facts about menopause, which they had gone to great lengths to obtain. Whatever your source of information, you probably have a fairly good understanding of the physiology, possible symptoms, and general happenings of menopause. Still, let's just cover a few of the basics.

Menopause is the time of life when a woman's ovaries wind down and production of the hormones that have been pumping out with regularity for forty or more years slows down. For certain women, this is a smooth and relatively innocuous transition, but others find the ride somewhat bumpy, accompanied by any number of uncomfortable symptoms.

When the ovaries age or when they are removed in an operation, the female hormones—particularly estrogen—that keep the female body and brain functioning are no longer produced in the same amounts. In the absence of adequate quantities of estrogen, a woman may start to experience some of the following symptoms:

❖ anxiety
❖ backache
❖ depression
❖ difficulty sleeping
❖ discomfort or pain during intercourse
❖ dry skin
❖ dry vagina
❖ headaches
❖ hot flashes
❖ increased facial hair
❖ irritability

❖ itchy skin (as if insects are crawling on the skin)
❖ joint aches
❖ lack of sexual drive
❖ light-headedness
❖ loss of concentration
❖ mood swings
❖ muscle aches
❖ poor memory
❖ tiredness
❖ urinary stress incontinence

Menopausal symptoms often start a few years before a woman's periods stop altogether; during this time, referred to as **perimenopause**, the symptoms are at their most severe. Sometimes periods quit abruptly, but more commonly they are sporadic, wavering between heavy and light until they finally stop completely. When periods have ceased entirely for a year, a woman is said to have reached **menopause**. Symptoms vary from none to severe among individual women, and they may last from a few months to several years. The average age of menopause is around fifty, but it can range anywhere between ages thirty-five and fifty-nine.

Hot flashes are the most distressing symptom reported by women in Dr. Liew's practice. In mild cases, women report a wave of heat creeping up the trunk, neck, and face for a few minutes. Some also complain of severe sweating following a hot flash—this can occur twenty to thirty times a day. At night, these severely affected women have to change their pajamas or nightclothes a few times because of the sweats, and they are invariably unable to tolerate any blankets, whether it's summer or winter.

Another noted symptom is loss of libido (interest in sex), which can go hand in hand with dryness of the vagina, making intercourse uncomfortable and irritating. Often estrogen replacement alone is not enough to improve lack of sexual desire, but it definitely helps with vaginal lubrication, eases the symptoms of vaginitis, and decreases the risk of recurrent bladder infections.

Plant estrogens, when eaten regularly for a few months, can help moisten a dry vagina, making sex more comfortable. Other symptoms, such as mood swings, irritability, and insomnia, may also respond quite well to estrogen supplementation.

Some complaints, although listed as symptoms of "menopause syndrome," may be the result of other medical conditions that are totally unrelated to menopause, but do occur more frequently in middle-aged and older people.

## Menopause and Hormone Replacement Therapy

Every woman (if she lives long enough) eventually goes through menopause. Some women sail through this phase of their lives without any problems, but a significant number require varying degrees of intervention and possibly even medical help with the multiple complaints associated with this time of life.

**Hormone replacement therapy** (HRT) may be the only answer for a certain number of women going through menopause. For these women, symptoms such as unbearable hot flashes and night sweats, an uncomfortably dry vagina, and roller-coaster mood swings may be only alleviated by HRT. For those whose lives have been drastically altered and their quality of life greatly diminished, medical treatment may indeed be the best option. There is no reason to suffer unduly during the menopausal years. Also, it's well known that female hormones are inextricably linked to bone health, and thus HRT should be considered for those who are clearly at risk for osteoporosis. Recent research suggests that estrogen also enhances brain function and may be used to prevent and treat Alzheimer's disease in women. The benefits of HRT may outweigh the risks for a number of women, and it should be seriously considered.

*Benefits of* HRT

❖   treats unbearable symptoms of menopause (hot flashes, dry vagina)

❖ preserves the bones and prevents osteoporosis
❖ may reduce the incidence of heart attacks and stroke
❖ may prevent and treat Alzheimer's disease

But nothing works for everyone, and so it goes with HRT. Some women are unable to tolerate outside hormonal intervention in any form. It has been estimated that up to a third of women who start HRT discontinue it for one reason or another. One obvious reason for stopping treatment is the number of uncomfortable and unwanted side effects.

## Common Side Effects of HRT

❖ fluid retention
❖ headaches
❖ irregular vaginal bleeding
❖ irritability
❖ nausea
❖ sore breasts
❖ venous thrombosis
❖ weight gain

A significant number of women simply cannot take HRT because it is contraindicated. This means that they currently have medical conditions that could be worsened by the addition of hormones. If you suffer from any of the following, HRT is not for you.

## Contraindications of HRT

❖ deep venous thrombosis and/or pulmonary embolus
❖ endometriosis
❖ hormone-dependent cancers such as breast cancer, ovarian cancer, or endometrial (uterine) cancer
❖ impending surgery requiring immobilization
❖ liver disease
❖ undiagnosed vaginal bleeding
❖ uterine fibroids

Hormone replacement therapy during and after menopause greatly helps some women, but it's clearly not for everyone. Before you make the all-important decision to take or not take HRT, learn all you can about it, and know its risks as well as its benefits.

## Potential Risks of HRT

❖ aggravation of pre-existing hormone-dependent cancers

❖ deep venous thrombosis and/or pulmonary embolus

❖ increased risk of breast cancer

❖ increased risk of uterine cancer

At the time of writing, some menopause clinics were testing HRT in selected women who in the past had had breast cancer and were treated with chemotherapy or radiotherapy. Until such trials have been completed and it is quite certain that HRT does not increase the recurrence rate of breast cancer, the majority of doctors will advise their patients to avoid it, or will prescribe it only with written informed consent from their patients.

## Plant Hormones Lessen Menopausal Symptoms

A lowered estrogen level is said to be responsible for all the symptoms of menopause. While this is too simplistic an explanation of the entire anthology of menopause-related complaints, it is true that a number of disturbing feelings may accompany declining production of female hormones.

A host of researchers have noted that a common factor links women's diets in countries where women in midlife are free from menopause-related complaints. These women eat plant foods containing estrogenlike substances that augment natural estrogen in their bodies. Laboratory tests have also shown that estrogenlike substances in foods can, in fact, have a marked influence on women's hormone status and general health.

Certain plant foods, ingested in sufficient amounts, contain enough plant estrogen (phytoestrogens) to elevate hormonal levels and curtail menopausal symptoms. When estrogen levels are low, a daily dose of specific foods eaten at a meal or as a snack may provide just enough of a boost to ward off hot flashes, moisten vaginal tissue, and even out mood swings.

Food substances that simulate hormone activity in the body are called **phytohormones**, but in reality they aren't true hormones such as those produced naturally by our bodies. Phytohormones can affect estrogen activity directly, or they can provide precursors to substances that later promote estrogen activity. Phytohormones may have differing effects, depending on a woman's natural hormonal level at the time of ingestion. They can stimulate estrogen production if levels are too low, and they also can reduce hormone levels if they are too high. This property is referred to as **hormonal modulation**, and it is evident in herbs such as dong quai and panax ginseng. Phytoestrogens (particularly the subcategory known as isoflavones) compete with the body's natural estrogens by attaching themselves to estrogen receptor sites on cell surfaces when there is excessive amounts of estrogen in the body, thereby reducing the potent effect of naturally produced estrogens on sensitive tissues such as the breasts and uterus. In an estrogen-deficient state, when there are more empty estrogen receptor sites, phytoestrogens occupy the empty sites and behave like weak natural estrogens. Phytoestrogens can do this because their chemical structure closely resembles that of natural estrogens.

Literally hundreds of plants contain estrogenlike substances. Some foods contain more potent phytoestrogens than others. Studies have shown that soy, flaxseed, rye, clover, and chickpeas (garbanzo beans) are among those with the most potent hormone-like effects. The foods listed below contain one or more of the phytoestrogen groups, which are called **isoflavones**, **lignans**, and **coumestans**. This list is by no means complete; further research is being carried out all the time.

## How Phytoestrogens React in a Woman's Body

How phytoestrogens work is still somewhat perplexing. They appear to have contradictory effects in women's bodies, depending on one's age and how much estrogen the body makes naturally. When a woman's estrogen levels wane, as in menopause, phytoestrogens exert estrogenlike activity and raise the estrogen level in the body's tissues; paradoxically, when a premenopausal woman generates high levels of estrogen, these same phytoestrogens block some of the natural estrogen from entering the cells, thus protecting against unhealthy exposure. Not only can phytoestrogens treat menopausal symptoms that result from declining estrogen levels, they also may protect against breast and uterine cancers, which are thought be promoted by continuing exposure to high levels of estrogen.

It is thought that estrogenlike substances from plant sources bind to estrogen receptor sites within the body, thus reducing the effects of the low-estrogen state characteristic of menopause. Even though such proestrogenic activity is very weak (from $\frac{1}{400}$th to $\frac{1}{1,000}$th the strength of women's natural estrogen), the boost may be enough to circumvent symptoms.

Phytoestrogens' effect on female tissues depends on many factors: the two most obvious are the amount of estrogen a woman's body is already producing and the saturation of her receptor sites. If natural estrogen is sufficient or elevated, then phytoestrogens compete for status on the receptor sites. If they successfully replace the natural estrogen that our bodies make, they are thought to protect us from unhealthy levels of one type of estrogen, estradiol.

This information has helped to explain observational studies of postmenopausal Asian women, who have not only fewer menopausal symptoms but also a lower rate of breast cancer. Significant amounts of excreted phytoestrogen byproducts have been found in the urine of Asian women, from ten to 100 times more than in that of Americans. Indeed, some researchers consider urinary excretion of plant estrogens a better indication of the health benefits such as

# The Estrogen Food List

### ❖ Legumes ❖

alfalfa, black-eyed peas, chickpeas (garbanzo beans), green
or French beans, green peas, lentils, mung bean sprouts,
navy beans, peanuts, red beans (adzuki beans), red clover,
soybeans, soy sprouts, split or field peas

### ❖ Oils ❖

corn oil, flaxseed oil, olive oil, sesame oil, soybean oil,
sunflower oil, rapeseed oil (canola oil)

### ❖ Vegetables ❖

beets, bok choy, broccoli, cabbage, carrots, cucumbers,
garlic, green peppers, mushrooms, potatoes, pumpkin,
rhubarb, seaweeds, squash, sweet potatoes, yams

### ❖ Spices and Herbs ❖

black cohosh, cloves, dong quai, fennel, ginger, hops,
licorice, sage, tea, thyme, turmeric

### ❖ Seeds ❖

flaxseed, sesame seed, anise seed, pumpkinseed,
sunflower seed

### ❖ Fruits ❖

apples, cherries, grapes, olives, papayas, pears, plums,
pomegranates, prunes

### ❖ Cereals/Grains ❖

barley, corn, oats, rice, rye, wheat

reduction of cholesterol, blood pressure, and hot flashes than other types of laboratory tests. High urinary excretion of phytoestrogens suggests adequate consumption, bacterial transformation, and absorption of phytoestrogens. In other words, the amount of phytoestrogens present in the urine tends to predict how much you'll benefit from eating phytoestrogen-rich foods. (A minority of people, however, are unable to absorb or benefit from phytoestrogens despite eating large amounts of phytoestrogen-containing foods. These people are considered nonresponders.)

Studies on the incidence of breast, colon, and prostate cancers among Asians and residents of Western countries have suggested that the incidence of these cancers is linked to diet. Migrant Asian populations that adopt a Western diet—high in fats and low in vegetables and fiber—have a much higher incidence of these cancers than do the population in their native lands. A typical Asian diet includes thirty to 100 milligrams of phytoestrogens daily; the Japanese consume up to 200 milligrams of phytoestrogens per day. Europeans and Americans take in a paltry one to five milligrams of phytoestrogens daily.

## Properties of Soy Proteins

Phytoestrogens in general, but particularly those found in soy foods, contain specific hormonelike substances called **isoflavones**. This large class of compounds (there are well over 4,000) occurs naturally in plants and can be further subdivided into more specific types, including daidzein, genistein, formononetin, and biochanin A. One of these, **genistein,** is considered the most powerful within this class of isoflavones and seems to be generating the most interest among food scientists, especially for its role in cancer therapy. Many ongoing studies are evaluating exactly how it works in human health.

There is much to learn about isoflavones, but we know at this time that they are a prolific family with benefits that extend beyond boosting women's estrogen levels. Consider some of their varied properties:

- ❖ antibacterial
- ❖ antiviral
- ❖ antifungal
- ❖ anti-inflammatory
- ❖ antioxidant

These properties are important aids in our bodies' fight against harmful bacteria, viruses, and fungi, and thus isoflavone-containing foods help keep us in good health. Although our bodies call on the immune system and produce antibodies to fight invaders, we need all the help we can get, and natural foods help us stay in top shape. Isoflavones' antioxidant effects are especially beneficial when free radicals are overabundant in our bodies, causing the degeneration of body parts such as blood vessels and joints. Isoflavones, along with other antioxidants, wipe up the free radicals and thus prevent long-term damage to vital organs and systems.

Isoflavones are also thought to have the following effects:

- ❖ restricting the growth of tumors
- ❖ building bone
- ❖ lowering high blood pressure
- ❖ lowering total and low-density lipoprotein (LDL) cholesterol, otherwise known as the bad cholesterol for its artery-clogging properties
- ❖ controlling hot flashes

It must be noted that although recent studies have shown that isoflavones can help preserve bone density, isoflavones are not as effective in this regard as the estrogens used in HRT. Most of these studies were done on animals, and the majority of those that focused on humans were short-term. More human studies, of longer duration, are now being carried out in Western countries. Their results will hopefully confirm what population studies have already implied: that humans consuming large amounts of phyto-estrogen-containing foods have lower osteoporotic fracture rates, thus emphasizing the osteoporosis-prevention effects of phyto-estrogens.

Animal studies have shown that genistein in particular does inhibit bone breakdown in the body, thus maintaining the animals' bone density. Ipriflavone (a synthetic isoflavone) has been shown to maintain bone density in postmenopausal women, and it also slows bone density loss in women whose ovaries have been removed.

## Studies on Soy and Hot Flashes

Is it possible that the natural estrogen diet will ever replace HRT as a way to curb menopausal symptoms? While the diet may not work for women with horrendous symptoms, there is evidence that it can effectively minimize hot flashes—among other symptoms—in moderate cases.

Isoflavones, which are found primarily in soy products, are basic to the Asian diet, and they are thought to be responsible for many health benefits specific to women. It has been estimated that the daily Asian diet may contain up to fifty grams of these soy proteins, as well as significant amounts of legumes, cereals, and grains, which are also rich in plant estrogens. Most experiments or trials use pure extracts of a particular isoflavone, but some studies have used or are now using soy flour or, more commonly, soy products to assess the effects of soy on blood pressure, cholesterol, hot flashes, and vaginal cell changes.

At the Second International Symposium on the Role of Soy in Preventing and Treating Chronic Disease (held in Brussels, Belgium, in September 1996), researchers looked at six human studies to determine the role of soy in reducing menopausal symptoms, especially hot flashes. While all six studies found at least a slight decline in the rate of hot flashes, three found a significant drop.

One of these studies, conducted in Melbourne, Australia, showed a 40 percent reduction in hot flashes when women consumed forty grams of soy flour each day for twelve weeks. Similar results were found in the United Kingdom (using eighty grams of isoflavones for two months) and in Italy (using sixty milligrams of isolated soy protein with seventy-six milligrams of isoflavones).

Continued research in the U.S.A. in 1998 adds credence to the theory that phytoestrogens—specifically those found in soy—can ease menopausal hot flashes. In a double-blind, placebo-controlled study, over 100 postmenopausal women, ages forty-eight to sixty-one, were divided into two groups. Each day for three months, one group was given an inert nonsoy tablet (a placebo), and the other was given sixty grams of isolated soy protein. The number of hot flashes and night sweats experienced by the women getting the soy was reduced by 45 percent by the end of the twelve weeks, compared to 30 percent in the placebo group.

It must be noted that some studies of soy's effects find no significant relief from hot flashes when the treatment group is compared to the nontreatment group. This suggests several things. First, it suggests that the placebo effect is very strong; in other words, women in the nontreatment groups felt better simply because that was what they'd expected. Secondly, it suggests that some women may be more sensitive to soy than others; finally, it suggests that the dosages in some of the studies were not adequate to elicit a response. It is also possible that women in the nontreatment groups may have consumed foods containing other plant estrogens that had been overlooked in the studies.

## How Much Soy Is Needed to Relieve Menopausal Symptoms?

No minimum daily requirement has been established for soy intake (or isoflavone content, as it is sometimes expressed). But the studies that have been conducted do provide clues as to what amount effectively reduces menopausal symptoms.

According to Loma Linda University soy pioneer and expert Mark Messina, Ph.D., the Japanese diet includes thirty to fifty milligrams of isoflavones on the average, which translates into about ten to twenty-five grams of soy protein ingested per day. To help you convert figures between soy intake and isoflavone content, consider that soy products contain roughly one to three milligrams of isoflavones per gram of protein. To put this into more practical terms, one serving of soy contains, on average, between four and twelve grams of soy protein, or twelve to forty-five milligrams of isoflavones

A serving of soy is considered a half-cup of tofu, tempeh, dry roasted soy nuts, or green soybeans, or one cup of soy milk. The goal should be about fifty milligrams of isoflavones per day or two servings of soy, depending on the food's isoflavone content. We recommend that you not eat all the soy at one time; instead, spread it out among your meals and snacks. The half-life of soy isoflavones is eight to twelve hours, and the level of isoflavones in your blood drops by half during this time. You'll get optimal results if you eat plant estrogens throughout the day.

It's not always easy to find out how much isoflavone is in the products you have chosen. Isoflavone levels in the soybean itself vary, and different brands of soy foods have different levels of isoflavones, so there are wide discrepancies among otherwise similar foods. Many food companies now offer isoflavone content information on their packages, but due to these variables, you should recognize that the information may not be exact.

Many factors determine the phytoestrogen levels of soy foods and of other foods that we eat, and other variables determine how much phytoestrogen our bodies can absorb. These are outlined in the next section.

## Factors Affecting Natural Phytoestrogens

❖ The season in which a plant is harvested is important in establishing its phytoestrogen content. Asians traditionally have been fussy about the timing of the harvest of plant and animal products. This knowledge is passed on from generation to generation, even though it is not generally accompanied by a scientific explanation. It is now known that concentrations of phytoestrogens vary with the maturity of the plant and the timing of its harvest.

❖ The genetic origin of the plant, and the climatic and environmental conditions under which it grew, also affect its phytoestrogen levels. For example, drought causes plants' phytoestrogen concentrations to increase. Genetic alteration of plants such as soy also affects phytoestrogen content.

❖ Processing of plant foods also affects phytoestrogen levels— the more a plant is processed, the lower its phytoestrogen content.

Even if a plant food's phytoestrogen levels are high, individual factors may affect how well the phytoestrogens are absorbed by our bodies:

❖ Appropriate bacteria must be present in the intestines of the consumer in order to properly digest and absorb phyto-estrogens.

❖ The transit time of the plant product in the intestines deter-mines how much phytoestrogen can be absorbed. Absorption depends on a normal and efficient gastrointestinal system.

## Other Natural Remedies That Regulate Hormonal Status

We can minimize the transitory symptoms of menopause by sim-ply changing our dietary and lifestyle habits. These changes include incorporating soy and other phytoestrogen-rich foods into our diets, but there are other steps we can take as well. Following are some of the suggestions outlined in Linda Ojeda's book *Menopause Without Medicine*.

❖ A **high-fiber diet** promotes the excretion of estrogen. Some women produce too much estrogen, and thus are at risk for estrogen-based cancers. A diet that includes twenty to forty grams of fiber a day binds with estrogen in the intestinal tract and helps remove it from the body.

❖ **Bioflavenoids** are compounds with structural and chemical similarities to estrogen, and they help to regulate estrogen levels in much the same way as phytoestrogens. They have been shown to control hot flashes, mood swings, anxiety, and heavy bleeding. Bioflavenoids are found in citrus fruits, grapes, cherries, cantaloupes, tomatoes, green peppers, and rose hips.

❖ A **low-fat diet**, with fats between 25 and 30 percent of total caloric intake, limits production of estrogen and encourages the excretion of excess estrogen.

❖ **Vitamin E**, which is essential for the production of sex hormones, effectively reduces menopausal symptoms such as hot flashes, vaginal dryness, and mood swings, and protects against heart disease and cancer. It's found in oil, nuts, seeds, sweet potatoes, and wheatgerm. Results are more effective with supplements in doses between 100 and 400 IU (international units), because the amount of vitamin E we receive from food is not adequate to minimize symptoms or protect us from heart disease and cancer.

❖ The essential fatty acids found in **flaxseed** act as weak estrogens in the body and thus help to keep all the tissues in the body well lubricated, including the skin, hair, and vaginal lining. These essential fats have been shown to reduce symptoms of menopause if they are ingested in doses of twenty-five grams (one to two tablespoons) per day.

❖ **B-vitamins** are instrumental in regulating estrogen in the body. When the Bs are insufficient, estrogen levels escalate. B-vitamins are founds in whole grains, beans, peas, chicken, and beef.

❖ **Boron** can mimic and enhance the action of estrogen and is needed to aid in calcium metabolism. Boron is found abundantly in fruits and vegetables, nuts, and flaxseed.

# CHAPTER TWO

## Plant Hormones and Other Health Concerns for Women

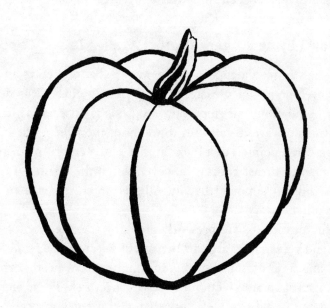

U p to this point in the book, we've been discussing the ways in which we can augment falling estrogen levels in menopause in order to stave off uncomfortable symptoms and possibly protect ourselves from heart disease and cancer. However, it's important to note that while most menopausal women experience declining estrogen levels, some *premenopausal* women are far from deficient in this female hormone. In fact, many women make more estrogen than they need. This may be due to heredity or to diet and lifestyle.

Over a lifetime, overexposure to estrogen can contribute to estrogen-based cancers of the breast and uterus. The information provided in this chapter explains how phytoestrogen-containing foods may help to fend off such cancers and also details the other, numerous benefits that these foods can offer both premenopausal and menopausal women. Hopefully, those women who have not yet reached menopause will be open to dietary and lifestyle changes that can benefit their future health.

## How Phytoestrogens Protect Against Breast Cancer

There is strong epidemiological evidence that diet plays a role in the development of breast cancer. This hypothesis was derived from population and migration studies that observed the food selections of various cultures throughout the world. The bulk of this research pointed to a high-fat diet as the culprit predisposing a woman to breast cancer; however, when the results of a large study did not support that hypothesis, interest began to focus upon other dietary factors.

Phytoestrogens are presently grabbing the attention of scientists and researchers around the world because diets containing high amounts of specific phytohormones have been correlated with a substantial reduction in breast cancer risk. For example, in a case-controlled study of more than 600 premenopausal women in Singapore, it was found that those who consumed the most soy were less likely to develop breast cancer than those who rarely touched it. Soy, the major source of isoflavones, seems to lengthen the menstrual cycle by one to five days, thus reducing the cells' exposure to estrogen and cutting the risk of breast cancer. Asian women are known to have longer menstrual cycles than Western women, as well as a lower risk of breast cancer.

Another case-control study, conducted in Australia by Dr. David Ingram and published in the *Lancet* in 1997, likewise found an association between phytoestrogen intake (as measured by urinary excretion) and the risk of breast cancer. After adjusting for possible confounding factors, such as age, parity, and alcohol and fat intake, the researchers noted a substantial reduction in breast cancer risk. This reduction, they felt, was unlikely to result from mere chance.

It is generally accepted that when estrogen levels stay too elevated for too long, a woman's risk of breast cancer increases. Reducing the effect of estrogen, it is widely believed, can produce a four- to five-fold reduction in breast cancer. One way to curtail estrogen production is to block the body's estrogen receptors before they can be filled with the strongest form of estrogen, **estradiol**. Specific isoflavones in soy, called **genistein** and **daidzein**, attach to the receptors in the breast and block estradiol, which is known to stimulate cancer cells in the breast. Two popular anticancer prescription drugs, tamoxifen and raloxifene, work the same way, although tamoxifen stimulates uterine cells at the same time; phytoestrogens do not adversely affect uterine cells. Indeed, plant estrogens appear to exert a positive influence on uterine cells, and thus phytoestrogen-containing foods have been studied in relation to another frightening female cancer, uterine cancer. Mark Goodman and his team at the Cancer Research Center of Hawaii studied 332 women of many different ethnic backgrounds and compared them to a control group. At the end of the study, the researchers found that the women who ate the most phytoestrogen-rich foods, including tofu and beans, had a 54 percent reduction in the risk of uterine cancer.

Soy and flaxseed, another phytoestrogen-rich food, contain yet another family of plant components, called **lignans**, that are thought to reduce both estrogen exposure and cancer risk. Lignans are a type of fiber that is changed by friendly bacteria in the gut into compounds that fight against cancer. Lignans have a biochemical structure similar to that of isoflavones and women's own natural estrogen, and thus they are able to fill estrogen receptors and thwart normal estrogen activity. Studies have shown that women who have breast cancer excrete lower amounts of lignans than do healthy women.

Lignans are structural components of plants such as fruits, legumes, vegetables, and grains, but they are found in greatest concentration in flaxseed (not the oil, just the seeds). The National Cancer Institute is looking at flaxseed as a potential cancer-fighter because it houses both lignans and **omega-3 fatty acids**, a healthy type of fat that shrinks cancer tumors and has a potent effect on breast, prostate, and lung cancer cells.

No one is saying that soy and flaxseed alone are going to cut your risk of cancer. But evidence suggests that one or two daily portions of soy and a tablespoon of flaxseed, along with other cancer-fighting nutrients and lifestyle changes, may reduce your risk. Since such a regimen causes no harm to the body—and indeed brings benefits—and since there is at least a chance that it might reduce your cancer risk, why not give it a try?

## Other Ways to Slow Down Estrogen Production in the Breast

### Pay Attention to the Kind of Fats You Eat

The kind of fat you eat is more important than the amount of fat in your diet. A classic study of 350,000 women in 1996, reported in the *New England Journal of Medicine*, debunked the theory that a high-fat diet increased the risk of breast cancer. After one sifts through the research, it becomes clear that the type of fat, rather than merely the amount of fat, that women eat can possibly promote or prevent breast cancer.

| Fats to Avoid |
| --- |
| **Saturated fats**—found in red meats and whole-fat dairy products like milk, butter, cheese, and creams |
| ***Trans* fatty acids**—found in margarine, fried foods, crackers, cookies, and bakery products |
| **Polyunsaturated oils**—safflower oil, corn oil, soybean oil, peanut oil, and sesame oil |

According to the current scientific literature, the safest oils are believed to be olive oil and canola oil, two monounsaturated oils. A recent Swedish study of over 60,000 women reported that monounsaturated fat reduced the risk of breast cancer by 45 percent. Two tablespoons per day in place of other fats is recommended.

Oils from fresh fish are an easy way to cut down on the body's excess estrogen. The omega-3 fatty acids found in coldwater fish (such as salmon, mackerel, and herring) and in cod liver oil can actually reduce tumors in lab tests and in studies on animals and humans. Many scientific journals have published accounts of omega-3 fatty acids being used in supplement form to treat various cancers. Don't overdo it; unless you are under the care of a physician, we do not advise megadosing with any supplement, including omega-3 fatty acids. However, choosing fish for dinner a few times a week and using olive or canola oil in your cooking are safe ways to provide the healthy fats your body needs.

### Maintain a High-Fiber Diet

A diet that includes plenty of fiber enhances excretion of estrogen from the body. One study showed that Finnish women who ate a high-fat diet but also incorporated adequate daily fiber had two-thirds the incidence of breast cancer of Western women.

Fiber may also bind with and dispose of carcinogens that we ingest in foods and absorb from the environment, making it doubly protective. Women who eat whole grains, beans, and fruits and vegetables are rarely constipated, and it appears that there is a relationship between constipation and breast disease. Women who have two or fewer bowel movements per week experience four times the incidence of breast disease of women who have them once a day.

Recommended daily fiber amounts range between thirty and forty grams. High-fiber cereals and legumes are your best sources.

## Keep Your Body Fat Moderate to Low

Excess body fat means excess estrogen. Body fat encourages estrogen production, and too much estrogen makes it very easy for the body to store fat, and thus a vicious cycle begins. If you are already overweight, it is not easy to stop this cycle, especially if you are older and if you have dieted and regained your weight several times. Losing weight slowly through exercise and limiting calories (particularly by not eating large amount of carbohydrates—sugars and starches—at one sitting) works for most women. Whatever you do, do not go on an ultra-low-fat diet. (In other words, don't let your fat intake fall below 15 percent of your daily calories. The optimal level of fat intake is between 20 percent and 30 percent of total calories.) Such diets are not effective for most women, and they rob you of essential fats and fat-soluble vitamins.

## Try Cruciferous Vegetables

Vegetables from the cabbage family—which includes cabbage, broccoli, bok choy, brussels sprouts, cauliflower, kale, turnips, radishes, and watercress—play a role in curtailing the formation of cancer cells. An ingredient called **indole 3-carbinol** turns estrogen into another substance less harmful to the body. Also found in such vegetables are many sulfur-containing compounds; one class of these compounds, called **glucosinolates**, has also shown anti-cancer properties.

## Be Cautious with Alcohol

Alcohol causes estrogen levels to rise. Even light to moderate drinking slows down the burning of fats, making it easy to store fat on the body. Couple drinking with eating high-fat foods, and you have a recipe for obesity. If you are already overweight (and thus overproduce natural estrogen), alcohol may have an even more damaging effect. Heavy drinkers (women who drink more than four glasses of alcohol per day) increase their chances of getting breast cancer by more than 40 percent.

## Women, Heart Disease, and HRT

Most women fear breast cancer more than heart disease, yet nearly twice as many women die from heart disease and stroke than from all forms of cancer combined. While 2.5 million American women are hospitalized for cardiovascular disease each year (of these, 500,000 die), women remain in the dark about what is taking their lives.

Women may not realize that heart disease is a different experience for women than for men. Women are less likely than men to be diagnosed with heart disease, and women are less likely to recover from it. Medications and medical interventions that save men's lives may not be as effective for women. Even the diet that has been proposed as the standard heart diet may not be appropriate for women. (For the full report on women and heart disease, read *Her Healthy Heart*, by Linda Ojeda.)

One of HRT's major marketing claims is that it protects against heart disease. But if this is your primary reason for turning to hormones, you may want to reconsider.

A landmark study, the Heart and Estrogen Progestin Replacement Study (HERS), found that postmenopausal women with existing coronary heart disease received no benefit from HRT. This study, which was the first randomized, controlled trial of HRT, was published in the *Journal of the American Medical Association* on August 19, 1998. The researchers recommended that women with coronary heart disease should not take HRT solely as a hedge against heart disease. The study also confirmed earlier findings that the hormone preparation produced higher rates of gallbladder disease, increased blood clotting in the legs and lungs, and raised levels of triglycerides (a type of unhealthy fat that can harm the heart).

## Soy Protects the Heart

Incorporating soy into your diet may be a preferable alternative to HRT. Eight decades of accumulated evidence indicate that soy protein significantly affects blood cholesterol and strengthens the heart in several ways. An exhaustive meta-analysis of thirty-eight studies examining the effect of soy protein on serum lipid (blood fat) levels showed the following average reductions in cholesterol:

❖ Total cholesterol declined 23.2 mg/dl (9.3 percent).

❖ LDL cholesterol dropped 21.7 mg/dl (12.9 percent).

❖ Triglycerides declined 13.3 mg/dl (10.5 percent).

The authors of this comprehensive review of the literature stated that soy can reduce the risk of coronary heart disease by 18 to 28 percent. Specifically, their analysis indicated the following:

❖ A daily intake of 25 grams of soy protein over several months could reduce blood cholesterol by 8.9 mg/dl.

❖ An intake of 50 grams of soy protein could reduce it by 17.4 mg/dl.

❖ An intake of 75 grams could reduce it by 26.3 mg/dl.

If a low-fat diet has not lowered your cholesterol levels, try soy. In a study at the University of Illinois, sixty-six postmenopausal women with cholesterol readings above 200 mg/dl were divided into two groups. Half followed a low-fat diet, using nonfat milk as the protein source, and the other half were given soy. Both groups experienced a reduction in total cholesterol; however, only the soy group saw a significant reduction in LDLs plus a rise in HDLs (see the glossary in the back of the book for a discussion of these two terms). However, the researchers noted that such results are seen in women with high cholesterol levels. If your cholesterol levels fall within the average range, you probably won't notice any change.

Soy proteins have several antiatherogenic (heart-healthy) effects in addition to lowering cholesterol. Consider the following.

❖ Soy isoflavones, phytates, and saponins have strong antioxidant activity and help curb the formation of toxic free radicals, which contribute to arterial damage.

❖ There is some evidence that genistein, the principal phytoestrogen in soy, may work in the early stages of atherosclerosis (a condition that leads to clogged arteries, diminished blood flow, and possibly heart failure) by hindering the overgrowth of epithelial cells lining the arteries. Such overgrowth promotes plaque buildup and clogged arteries.

❖ Genistein also appears to prevent blood clots, which can lead to heart attack and stroke, by inhibiting the formation of an enzyme called thrombin.

❖ Genistein may increase the flexibility of blood vessels, helping to prevent spasms that can trigger a heart attack.

❖ Soy has a modulating effect on blood sugar levels. Glycine and arginine, the amino acids in soy, decrease insulin levels in the blood, thus tempering blood sugar levels. Keeping blood sugar fairly stable is important for women, because the combination of high estrogen levels and high insulin levels has a doubly negative effect on both the heart and breasts.

## Other Heart-Healthy Strategies

❖  Cut down or eliminate saturated fats (found in red meats and whole-fat dairy products), *trans* fatty acids (found in margarine, hydrogenated bakery products, and fried foods), and polyunsaturated oils (safflower, corn, and sunflower oil). All three negatively affect blood cholesterol levels and make women more vulnerable to heart disease.

❖  Fats that hold the favored stamp of approval include the monounsaturated oils, olive and canola. They have potent antioxidant properties that fend off artery damage from LDL cholesterol, and they've been shown to reduce LDLs without lowering HDLs. The marine omega-3 fatty acids (which are found in fish) show great promise for keeping hearts healthy. A study at the University of Washington, which looked at both women and men, found that those who reported eating one serving of fatty fish a week had half the risk of heart attacks of those who shunned fish.

❖  Don't go too low with your fats. In a report in the September 1, 1998, issue of *Circulation*, the American Heart Association stated that very-low-fat diets may not provide additional benefits for the heart. The report, which summarized several clinical studies, indicated that cutting fat to less than 15 percent of total daily calories may lower beneficial HDLs and raise triglycerides, changes that are thought to raise heart disease risk. The optimal level of fat intake for heart health is between 20 and 30 percent of total calories.

❖  Soluble fiber, as found in oat bran, beans, legumes, apples, carrots, and whole grains, promotes the excretion of cholesterol and lowers both total and LDL cholesterol. It improves sugar metabolism, reduces blood insulin levels, and delays the emptying of the stomach, producing a feeling of fullness that can be useful if you wish to lose weight.

According to the Harvard School of Public Health, omitting fiber from your diet is just as important a risk factor for heart disease as cigarette smoking, high blood cholesterol, and high blood pressure. Your total daily fiber goal should be thirty to forty grams; of that, one-third of the total (twelve grams) should be soluble fiber. Sources of soluble fiber include the following:

### 2 *to* 3 *grams*:

Up to 1 cup bran and oat cereals (depending on brand)

½ cup cooked kidney beans

1 large apple

½ cup brussels sprouts

### A*bout* 1 *gram*:

Up to 1 cup other cereals

½ cup cooked split peas

1 carrot

3 dried prunes

¾ cup asparagus

❖ Flaxseed lowers cholesterol. Flaxseed is the primary source of healthy omega-3 fatty acids in the plant kingdom. While flaxseed oil is not as potent as the fat of coldwater fish, it does provide unique benefits that set it apart and establish it as a superb fat for the heart. Another essential fatty acid (EFA) found in flaxseed, alpha linolenic acid, may protect against stroke. This particular EFA can reduce the "stickiness" of the blood's platelets, thus preventing dangerous blood clots from forming. Flaxseed is also a fair source of both soluble and nonsoluble fiber (an eighth of a cup offers ten grams of fiber). It houses lignan precursors that are converted by bacteria during digestion into phytoestrogens. Because of any one or all of these factors, flaxseed has been shown to lower cholesterol between 5 and 15 percent. Various studies on flaxseed have used amounts between five and fifty grams to effect changes in blood fats.

❖ An array of antioxidants, such as vitamins C and E, beta carotene, and a host of others, guard against heart disease by preventing LDL cholesterol from oxidation by free radicals. Although the list of studies on the benefits of individual antioxidants seems endless, an important study out of Harvard University has demonstrated that these potent health-protecting nutrients work best in combination. Women who took vitamin E and C and beta carotene on a regular basis experienced a remarkable decrease in heart disease risk—50 percent—and their stroke rate fell 54 percent.

To get a healthy dose of antioxidants, we should eat two to three servings of fruit and four to five servings of vegetables per day. Because few people manage to eat the requisite number of servings, a multivitamin/mineral tablet taken as a supplement may be necessary—note that supplements should be used as an adjunct to these wonderful fruits and vegetables, not as a replacement for them.

❖ Getting enough of three B-vitamins—folic acid and vitamins B-6 and B-12—should be a major concern for anyone at risk for heart disease. When any one of the trio is lacking, homocysteine levels may rise in the blood. Homocysteine is a normal substance in the blood, but when it is elevated, it is considered one of the top risk factors for heart disease. In July 1997, The New England Journal of Medicine uncovered more than seventy-five clinical and observational studies that demonstrated a relationship between high homocysteine levels and coronary artery disease, peripheral artery disease, and stroke.

Researchers from the Harvard School of Public Health have proposed the theory that homocysteine damages the arteries' inner lining, beginning a process that fosters the proliferation of epithelial cells and plaque buildup. Other researchers have suggested that homocysteine seems to thicken the blood and may also facilitate the oxidation of LDL cholesterol.

Menopausal women are particularly at risk, because when estrogen wanes, homocysteine rises. To ensure that you get 400 micrograms of folic acid each day, breakfast on a bowl of folic acid–fortified cereal, lunch on a bowl of lentils, and snack on a variety of fruits and vegetables. If this doesn't sound doable, consider taking multivitamin and mineral tablets, which offer the requisite amount of folic acid as well as moderate amounts of vitamins B-6 and B-12. We recommend a vitamin tablet containing between twenty and fifty micrograms of both vitamins B-6 and B-12.

❖ Garlic has been reported to lower total cholesterol by 15 to 20 percent, to lower LDLs and triglycerides, and to increase HDLs. It reduces blood pressure and blunts the blood's clotting tendency (clotting can lead to heart attacks). Incorporating garlic into your cooking, using it as an accompaniment to vegetable dishes, or offering it as an appetizer, along with the other dietary guidelines outlined in this book, may ward off a heart attack as well as any lurking vampires.

❖ Modern science has confirmed what early Egyptian writings noted about onions: they are a tonic for the blood. Scientific literature has reported that onions inhibit the formation of fibrinogen, which is a substance that the body produces to ensure proper blood clotting, especially when injury occurs. Thus onions can help to break up and dissolve potentially dangerous clots. Harvard cardiologist Dr. Victor Gurewich found in his practice that taking the juice of a single onion daily raised HDL levels about 70 percent of the time.

❖ Green tea possesses important polyphenols, which are yet another group of phytochemicals that possess potent antioxidant properties. Substitute green tea for your morning coffee or late afternoon pick-me-up.

## Hormones Prevent Bone Loss

It is well known that both estrogen and progesterone help preserve women's bone density, and as a result millions of American women take HRT to protect against bone loss, which leads to osteoporosis. Estrogen prevents the bone loss that accompanies menopause. It does not reverse already established osteoporosis, but it does stop natural or accelerated bone deterioration. Doctors recommend that HRT continue indefinitely if it is to be successful.

Fortunately, low-dose estrogen preparations (0.3 milligrams) have been found to be as effective in preventing bone loss as the standard 0.625-milligram formulation. It's quite possible that a lower dosage also causes fewer side effects, so it may be tolerable for women who were forced to discontinue their treatment due to uncomfortable side effects. It is still unknown whether a lower dosage lessens the risk for breast cancer. However, it's always a promising advance when a lower dose of any medication achieves the same result.

Some studies suggest that progesterone is the more important female hormone in the battle against osteoporosis because it actually builds new bone. In what is now called a landmark study of progesterone, Dr. John Lee asked postmenopausal women with existing osteoporosis to apply a cream containing 3 percent progesterone to their skin for two weeks out of the month. He also advised them to follow specific dietary guidelines and take nutritional supplements. The study found that, among 100 patients who had serious bone loss, sixty-three experienced bone-density increases of 15.4 percent following the treatment. The expected bone-density loss for this age group is 4.5 percent.

Natural progesterone, as opposed to the synthetic progestins found in oral preparations, appears to be free of side effects. Conclusive research has yet to be done, but many nutritionally oriented doctors are prescribing natural progesterone and an even larger number of women are utilizing this approach. It is generally recommended that women apply one-quarter to one-half teaspoon of progesterone cream to their inner arms, abdomen, or inner thighs for two weeks out of the month. Because many of the natural progesterone products on the market contain very small amounts of the hormone, this book's Resources section lists a few that are reputable and contain known quantities of the hormone. You can also get information about these creams and their use from their manufacturers.

## Can Plant Hormones Protect Bones?

Researchers have still not determined with absolute certainty whether plant hormones are potent enough to prevent or arrest bone loss. It is known that the isoflavones genistein and daidzein are similar to synthetic estrogen, which is effective in preventing or retarding bone loss, but whether they can replace HRT is not yet known.

Early research found that isoflavones had a modest effect on bone tissue, but more recent studies appear more encouraging. Research conducted by John Anderson, of the University of North Carolina, showed that soy protein did prevent bone deterioration in rats whose ovaries had been removed, resulting in a diminished estrogen supply and attendant bone loss. When this group of rodents was compared to another group taking Premarin (the most common HRT medication, made from the urine of pregnant mares), the results showed that soy could prevent bone loss almost as well as synthetic hormones.

In a study on postmenopausal women, researchers from the University of Illinois compared sixty-six women who drank milk protein to a group of women who received soy protein that contained either fifty-six or ninety milligrams of isoflavones. The women who took soy protein with ninety milligrams of isoflavones every day for six months were found to have higher bone mineral density in their spines. Researcher Susan Potter found this encouraging but pointed out that the studies need to be extended over one to three years. The study also found that doses of isoflavones below 90 mg did not work.

A review covering published reports on population studies, lab cultures on cells and tissues, and experimental studies on animals concluded that taking isoflavones (especially genistein and daidzein) at optimal doses resulted in improved bone mass.

How much isoflavone should you take to treat and prevent bone loss? Experts have speculatively suggested that between sixteen and twenty grams of soy protein (which would provide sixteen to sixty milligrams of isoflavone) taken daily is sufficient for prevention. Practically, for those of us who think in terms of servings of a food, this means one to two servings of soy per day. For treatment, the studies used ninety milligrams of isoflavones, which means that you would have to double the servings of soy per day. Many women may find this impractical and would rather take their chances with HRT. But what should women do if they cannot take HRT? Drugs that appear to preserve bone are currently available, and you may consider discussing them with your doctor.

If you are determined to use natural methods but cannot incorporate this amount of soy into your diet, don't get discouraged. Remember that soy is but one of many ways to keep the bones healthy. In fact, we should all remember that soy foods and medication should be combined with other bone-building practices in order to be effective. The next section outlines some of these practices.

## A Lifestyle Program to Build Bones

Soy and other estrogen-rich foods may spare you further bone loss, so it makes sense to include these foods in your anti-osteoporosis diet. However, a complete bone-healthy program should also include the following:

❖ Stop smoking. Female smokers lose bone mass faster than nonsmokers, probably because the associated drop in estrogen may diminish absorption of calcium.

❖ Limit caffeine. Excess intake is associated with increased urinary excretion of calcium.

❖ Limit sodas. They are high in phosphoric acid, which interferes with your intestinal calcium absorption and urinary excretion.

❖ Your basic diet should be high in carbohydrates, relatively low in fat, and low in meat proteins. Red meat is very high in phosphorus, a mineral that in high doses leaches calcium from the bones.

❖ Keep your alcohol intake moderate. Too much alcohol causes calcium to be poorly absorbed and interferes with vitamin D metabolism.

❖ Make certain you get the full supply of bone-building nutrients:

**Calcium** is critical to bone health. The National Institutes of Health suggest that women up to age fifty, as well as postmenopausal women on HRT, should get 1,000 milligrams daily. For postmenopausal women not on HRT, 1,500 milligrams is recommended. Good food sources include low-fat yogurt and milk, tofu made with calcium sulfate, almonds, fortified cereals, and leafy green vegetables.

**Magnesium** deficiency may weaken bones as much as inadequate calcium. A study at Purdue University found that menopausal women given magnesium hydroxide for two years saw a significant increase in bone density. Your daily magnesium intake should be between 500 and 800 milligrams per day. Dietary surveys have shown that up to 85 percent of

American women consume less than the recommended daily allowance (RDA).

**Vitamin D**, the sunshine vitamin, is needed to absorb calcium. Women should take in about 400 IU (international units) per day. A thirty-minute walk in the sun, if your skin is exposed, provides about 300 IU.

**Boron**, the mineral found in nuts, beans, fruits, and vegetables, helps raise levels of blood estrogens in postmenopausal women, which may help them to retain calcium. Taking a three-milligram boron supplement daily has been shown to reduce calcium excretion by 44 percent. If you regularly eat your fruits and veggies, supplements aren't necessary.

Many other nutrients affect calcium absorption and bone health. Consider some of the lesser-known vitamins and minerals that protect the bones: Vitamin C, K, and the minerals manganese and copper.

❖ Exercise. Bone density depends on how much the bone is stressed. Women on estrogen who do not exercise, do not gain bone mass. Weight-bearing exercises such as walking, dancing, and weight training, done for thirty minutes three times a week, strengthen your bones, heart, and entire body.

# CHAPTER THREE

✛

# An Introduction to Soy

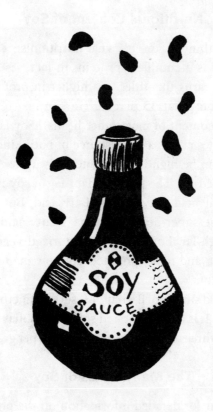

Not too long ago, soy products were found only in Asian markets and health-food stores, but given their glowing promise for a variety of health concerns, they are worming their way onto the shelves of local supermarkets. Once nondescript oddities, soy products are now manufactured with American tastes in mind, and the variety of soy-based foods is expanding every year. Still, habits are slow to change, and we are often reluctant to try foods that have been foreign to our diets for so long. This chapter will introduce you to the ever-increasing choices in soy, but before we begin, it is important to understand why soy is considered such a superb food and why we encourage you to make it a regular part of your diet.

## Nutritional Content of Soy

Soy is loaded with nutrition. It's what nutritionists call a nutrient-dense food. Soy is a complete protein; in fact, it's the only vegetable food that earns this title. It is higher in protein than other legumes, weighing in at 35 percent (in contrast to the 20 to 30 percent protein content of most other beans). Soy is high in complex carbohydrates and is a good source of both kinds of fiber.

While soy can be high in fat (sometimes up to 40 percent), it is low in saturated fat. The predominant fat in soy is the essential fatty acid linoleic acid, an omega-6 fatty acid. But soy also contains some of the super-healthy omega-3 fatty acids. Not all soy products are high-fat. For example, texturized vegetable protein (TVP) has no fat, and many products are now manufactured with a lower fat content.

Soy has a good supply of B-vitamins, several micronutrients, and phytochemicals. It is a concentrated source of isoflavones, containing about one to three milligrams of isoflavones per gram of protein.

## The Many Faces of Soy

See Chapter Four for detailed information on the protein, fat, and caloric content of soy foods.

## Soybeans

Soybeans belong to the legume family. The plant produces pods that, when mature, each contain two or three seeds. These seeds are the famous soybeans—sometimes called soya beans—which have been used in China for several thousand years. In China, the soybean is commonly known as *wang tul* or "yellow bean."

Dried soybeans are a yellowish to creamy color with a rather tough skin, and they're slightly smaller in size than green or garden peas. Soybeans can be purchased dried, like other beans, or fresh, as green soybeans. Either way, they contain about 35 percent protein by weight and are a good source of isoflavones, B-vitamins, calcium, and fiber. The down side is that soybeans are harder to find than some of the other soy products, and they are decidedly tougher than most other types of beans. Many people find the flavor on the strong side, so if it is not to your liking, choose other soy foods.

Dried soybeans can be boiled for several hours, like any other bean, and eaten as a side dish or added to salads or casseroles. Fresh green soybeans look like fuzzy green pods. When they are steamed until tender, they are sweet and crunchy and are a great addition to salads or can be eaten plain as a snack. Soybeans in the pod, known as *edamame,* can be found in stores, already cooked and ready to eat. Canned soybeans are also available. They can be easily served on toast or mixed into salads or casseroles.

## Soy Milk and Other Soy Drinks

Soy milk is a milklike liquid prepared from ground soybeans and water. It is lactose-free, and people who cannot digest the sugar in cow's milk often drink it as a substitute. Unfortified soy milk is packed with protein (about eight grams per cup, although this varies), B-vitamins, and isoflavones. It does not contain as much calcium as cow's milk, but like regular milk, it may be fortified with calcium, vitamin D, and, sometimes, vitamin B-12.

Manufacturers have made great strides in making soy milk palatable. No longer is it the grainy, beany drink of the past. Today soy milk is light and smooth, and it is sold plain and in a variety of flavors, including chocolate, almond, and vanilla. You can find it next to "real" milk in the refrigerated section of the market, or you can buy it packaged in aseptic quart containers or snack sizes that do not need refrigeration. Soy milk is also available in low-fat and nonfat varieties.

Soy milk is good enough to drink hot or cold; you can pour it over cereal or use it as a milk substitute in cooking.

## Soy Nuts

Soy nuts are dry-roasted or deep-fried soybeans that are normally flavored with salt or other seasonings. They're quick and tasty snacks, and they have the same nutritional qualities of the plain beans; however, they are high in fat and calories. Use them sparingly, in breads and baked goods.

## Miso

Miso is a fermented soybean paste that is made by mixing soybeans, salt, water, and a *koji* or cultured grain (usually rice or barley) as a starter. A tablespoon of miso has sixty to eighty calories and virtually no fat; however, it is quite high in sodium and should be used sparingly.

There are several types of miso, which vary in taste and usage depending on the color. Darker shades tend to be stronger and denser than the lighter varieties, which are normally sweeter and less salty. Miso can be used like bouillon to flavor soups; it can be added to sauces for vegetables and to salad dressings; and it can be used to marinate meat for barbecues.

Chinese and Southeast Asian stores sell miso in jars and packages. It will keep for up to a year if stored in an airtight container in the refrigerator.

## Tofu

Tofu or bean curd, as it is sometimes called, is made from soy milk. Dried soybeans are crushed and boiled and a curdling agent such as nigari or calcium sulfate is added to separate the curds from the whey. The pieces of the curds are then poured into square molds, where they become firm.

Tofu is a nutritional powerhouse. It's high in protein (a half-cup provides ten grams), it's rich in essential fats, and it's a good source of zinc, iron, B-vitamins, and calcium (if it is made with calcium sulfate). By itself, tofu has no flavor, so it's a natural additive to any healthy, tasty recipe.

Needless to say, tofu must be kept cool and consumed within two days of opening. A few companies now package tofu in aseptic containers that need no refrigeration and have a shelf life of ten months. See Resources, in the back of the book, for information.

You'll discover several forms of tofu in the refrigerated section of the market:

*Silken or soft tofu* has a creamy consistency and is best for soups, desserts, sauces, and some delicate dishes requiring a smooth texture. Blend it into drinks, puddings, and pureed vegetables.

*Firm tofu* handles cutting quite well and can be added to vegetable dishes, stews, chili, and casseroles.

*Hard tofu* can be deep-fried, marinated for barbecuing, and crumbled in salads or topping for pasta.

*Deep-fried tofu puffs* are small cubes of tofu, light brown in color. They are very light and airy inside and can be eaten straight from the package with a soy or chili sauce or added to soups, stews, and stuffings. They can also be cut up into smaller sizes and added to salads, much like croutons in a Caesar salad. Notice that they are deep-fried and thus should be used sparingly.

*Tofu desserts, mayonnaise, cream cheese, yogurt,* and *dips* are among some of the new products made with tofu. Some of these are wonderful substitutes for the traditional products. Do check the labels for fat content and other added ingredients. Just because it advertises itself as a tofu or soy product does not necessarily mean it is healthy.

## Soy Flour

Soy flour is made from the dehulled soybean, which is milled, toasted, and ground. Full-fat soy flour is very high in fat, so look for defatted flour, in which the oil has been extracted during processing. Defatted soy flour is not only lower in calories and fat than ordinary wheat flour, but is also higher in protein.

Soy flour is heavier than wheat flour and is creamy in color with a distinctive "beany" smell that usually translates into a rather nutty flavor after cooking. Cakes, biscuits, and cookies can be made from soybean flour, but you'll want to use it in combination with a lighter flour. To see how it works, try substituting about 20 percent of the wheat flour with soy flour in one of your tested favorite recipes (soy flour can substitute for between 30 and 50 percent of the regular flour in your recipes). You may need to add a bit more moisture if the dough seems too dry. Note that since soy flour typically browns more quickly than wheat flour, lowering baking temperature by twenty-five degrees may be necessary. Soy flour does not contain gluten, so you cannot substitute it entirely for wheat flour in yeast breads.

Because soy flour is gluten-free, it's a good alternative for individuals with celiac disease. Store soy flour in the refrigerator or freezer until you are ready to use it.

## Soy Sauce

Soy sauce is made from salted, roasted soybeans that have been fermented for a few months to a year in huge vats. It is said that the sauce tastes better if the container is made of wood.

There are basically two types of soy sauce, light and dark. Both types are used in Chinese cooking, while in several other nations, light soy is the only type widely used. The lighter soy sauce is normally used for marinating meat, fish, and poultry, and for making sauces. Dark soy sauce, which is thick and viscous from the inclusion of molasses, is reserved for richer stews and sauces. Generally, dark soy sauce is sweeter and less salty, and it gives meat a lustrous, dark-brown color. The manufacturer may add black beans to the processing; this is known as black-bean soy sauce. Mushrooms are sometimes added to the soy sauce extracts during processing, producing mushroom soy sauce. The soy sauce brands most commonly available in North American supermarkets (Kikkoman, La Choy, etc.) are light soy sauces. At Asian groceries in the U.S. you can obtain not only dark soy, but the more delicate-flavored light soys imported from China, Hong Kong, and Taiwan (brands such as Pearl River, Superior Soy, and Amoy). If there is no Asian market nearby, Tamari (a very rich Japanese soy sauce) is available at most health food stores and makes a passable substitute for dark soy. Add a generous pinch of sugar to any recipe in which you are substituting a light soy or Tamari for dark soy.

Soy sauce is low in isoflavones, so it's not considered a potent phytonutrient, as are the other soy products. It is high in salt and should be used sparingly, especially if you suffer from high blood pressure or kidney disorders. You can find low-salt versions; check the labels.

## Soybean Sprouts

This product must not be confused with mung bean sprouts, which are readily available in most supermarkets. Soybean sprouts, which you can buy in packages from Asian food stores and specialty stores, take longer to cook than mung bean sprouts. Their roots are slightly stringy, and the cotyledons (seed leaves) are very bright yellow in color and thick and broad in structure. This part of the sprout contains the most nutrients and gives it a very nutty taste.

Weight for weight, the phytoestrogen (coumestrol) content in soybean sprouts is at least fourteen times greater than that in alfalfa sprouts and seventy times greater than that in frozen green or string beans. Like the mung bean sprout, the soybean sprout is also a good source of vitamin C.

Both beans can be sprouted at home at your convenience. Should you care to experiment, purchase very fresh soybeans and presoak them in cold water overnight. Sow onto a supporting porous bed in a clean container and keep in an airy place away from direct sunlight. Water twice daily and drain the water so that the sprouting beans do not soak in water at all times. The bean sprouts will be ready to harvest in four days. Remove the skin before cooking. The sprouts can be kept for two days in the refrigerator after harvesting.

## Lecithin

Lecithin is a byproduct of soybean oil. It is a natural emulsifier used to manufacture a wide variety of products, such as candy, bakery products, chocolate coatings, and margarine. Lecithin is gaining popularity in the health field because of its antioxidant properties and potential cholesterol-lowering effect.

Lecithin is available in powdered and granular forms and in tablets, often combined with other vitamins and minerals. You can add the powder or granules to milk shakes, eggnogs, soups, and salads, or sprinkle them over your breakfast cereal.

## Soybean Oil

Soybean oil is an extract from soybeans. Although soybean oil does not contain isoflavones, it is rich in omega-3 and omega-6 fatty acids, as well as linolenic and linoleic acid, which are said to help prevent bowel and breast cancers. Oil derived from soy has a light, bland flavor and a high smoking point that makes it attractive for cooking or stir-frying vegetables, which requires high heat. Many commercial products are made with soybean oil, such as baked goods, prepared foods, and salad dressings.

## Tempeh

Tempeh is made from fermented soybeans, usually mixed with a grain such as rice or millet. It has a meatlike texture and tastes nutty, somewhat like a mushroom. Tempeh can be marinated for grilling or barbecuing. Chunks of tempeh can also be added to chili or spaghetti sauce, or pan-fried with mushrooms, onions, and bread crumbs for a delicious stuffing. It can be grated and made into vegetarian burgers or diced and added to salads.

Tempeh is a rich source of protein, fiber, isoflavones, iron, potassium, calcium, and B-vitamins, particularly vitamin B-12, which is usually found only in foods of animal origin.

## Soy Grits

Soy grits are made by removing the soybeans' skin prior to lightly steaming and grinding them. They taste much like soybeans and have a similar nutritional value. Because their texture is similar to ground beef, they are a good substitute in meat dishes such as chili, meat loaf, stew, casseroles, and spaghetti sauce.

## Texturized Soy or Vegetable Protein

TSP or TVP is compressed soy flour that is used to extend ground beef dishes such as meat loaf, chili, and hamburgers. TSP is an excellent source of soy protein (one ounce provides sixteen grams) and isoflavones. Its real bonus is that it has almost no fat. TSP products have varying levels of plant estrogens, depending on how they were processed. TSP must be rehydrated before using, and it keeps up to four days in the refrigerator once made.

## Other Soy Products

Every month seems to bring new and improved soy products to
the shelves of the supermarket and the advertisements in health
magazines. Soy cheeses are taking up residence alongside regular
cheeses. They look like cheese and come in a good selection, from
mild to red-pepper hot. Try them as a substitute in your recipes
for quiche, pizza, and lasagna, or just eat them as a snack on
crackers.

Soy protein can mimic a variety of meat foods, and they can
look, feel, and almost taste like the genuine item. Soy-based hot
dogs, sausage, and vegetarian hamburgers are creeping into local
markets. While these lookalikes are usually lower in fat than the
real thing, they are a poor source of isoflavones, and unless fortified they do not have the same nutritional content as the other,
purer soy products.

Check out some of the other varieties of soy: soy mayonnaise,
cookies, breads, crackers, yogurt, and smoothies.

# CHAPTER FOUR

✛

# Integrating Natural Estrogens Into Your Life

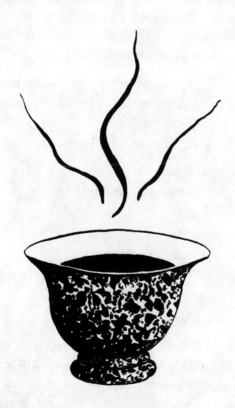

There are no official guidelines regarding natural estrogen intake in the daily diet, no recommended daily allowances or space allotted on the food pyramid. Official guidelines may be drawn up in the future as new scientific information becomes available and new standards are accepted. However, it may take another generation of scientists' work to steer us accurately through such a complicated maze. The following general recommendations are based on current knowledge derived from decades of research by various dedicated food scientists:

❖ For general good health, consume at least one or two servings of soy per day, aiming for total of thirty to fifty milligrams of isoflavones. On average, each gram of soy protein may contain one to three milligrams of phytoestrogens, as the genetic origin of the soy plants, their season of harvest, and the climatic and environmental conditions under which they were grown all influence phytoestrogen concentration.

Those who worry about fat content can look for fat-reduced varieties: in general, defatting of soy products does not significantly affect their phytoestrogen content.

Here are a few suggestions for serving sizes:

½ cup tofu or tempeh

3½ tablespoons soy protein powder

1 cup soy milk

½ cup cooked dried soybeans

½ cup dry roasted soy nuts

¼ cup TVP (reconstituted)

1 soy burger

2 soy hot dogs

❖ Consuming excessive amounts, such as four to five times the average Asian daily intake, is not necessarily more beneficial, as improvements in serum cholesterol, blood pressure, hot flashes, and other menopausal symptoms do not bear a linear relationship to your intake. Flooding all of your estrogen receptor sites with excessive phytoestrogens may actually produce an antiestrogenic response. So, eat in moderation.

❖ Make it a practice to eat different foods each day. A variety of foods are known to contain phytoestrogens, and those not yet tested may also contain these beneficial substances. Although grains, spices, fruits, and vegetables possess smaller amounts of phytoestrogens than soy, this does not mean they are ineffective, especially if many of these foods are ingested in the same day. In Asian diets, rice, barley, and other grains, seeds, beans, legumes, sprouts, tea, and seafood are featured in every meal. Vary your grains, fruits, and vegetables to get the most out of plant estrogens.

❖ Moderation with any food is best. Overindulgence in one particular foodstuff to the exclusion of other food groups can produce side effects. For example, an individual who eats excessive amounts of carrots, pumpkin, or corn can manifest carotenemia and turn orange; more importantly, in a young menstruating female, this condition can cause the cessation of periods (amenorrhea). Once the excess intake has stopped for a few months, normal function will resume.

❖ Broad-spectrum antibiotics kill friendly bacteria in the bowel, and therefore plant estrogens may not be available for absorption even though you've eaten adequate quantities of estrogen-rich foods. It may take two to six weeks for your system to recover after a course of antibiotics. Do not panic when hot flashes and menopausal symptoms reappear after a bout of antibiotics; it is only a temporary setback.

❖ Women experiencing sore breasts during the diet should avoid foods and beverages containing caffeine, as these tend to aggravate breast tenderness and lumpiness. If your periods are heavy, avoid foods containing high amounts of salicylates, such as tomatoes, oranges, and pineapples. Salicylates thin the blood and aggravate heavy menstrual flow. Resume your usual diet after a break of four to five days.

## General Health Guidelines

Some of the following information is repetitive; that's intentional. The basic pearls of wisdom bear repeating because we all have a penchant for forgetting the obvious.

The natural estrogen diet is primarily plant-based. Whether you choose to go vegetarian is up to you. Here are a few guidelines for establishing your own personal plan.

❖ *Whole grains*: seven to ten servings/day (one serving = half-cup grain, cereal, or pasta, or one slice bread)

❖ *Legumes*: seven or more servings/week (one serving = half-cup cooked beans)

❖ *Fruits*: two to three servings/day (one serving = one piece of fresh fruit, half-cup cooked fruit, or three-quarters cup fruit juice)

❖ *Vegetables*: three to four servings/day (one serving = half-cup cooked or one cup raw vegetables)

❖ *Soy foods*: one to two servings/day (one serving = one cup soy milk, half-cup tofu, tempeh, or green beans)

❖ *Meat, chicken, and fish*: no more than six ounces/day

❖ *Fiber*: A high-fiber diet helps to prevent breast cancer and maintain a healthy heart. Total per day should range between twenty-five and forty grams. The chart below shows the amount of fiber found in common foods.

| *Cereal*: |
| --- |
| ½ cup high-fiber cereal = 14 grams |
| ½ cup medium-fiber cereal = 8 grams |

**Beans:**

| | |
|---|---|
| ¾ cup of most beans = 14 grams | |
| 10 ounces split-pea soup = 4 grams | |

**Breads:**

| | |
|---|---|
| 1 slice whole wheat bread = 2 grams | |

**Fruit:**

| | |
|---|---|
| 1 medium apple = 4 grams | |
| 8 dried apricots = 3 grams | |
| 1 large banana = 2 grams | |

**Vegetables:**

| | |
|---|---|
| 1 large baked potato = 4 grams | |
| ½ cup cooked broccoli = 2 grams | |

❖ Keep total fats in your diet between 20 and 30 percent of total calories per day. If you are eating approximately 2,000 calories per day, this translates to forty-four to sixty-six grams of fat each day. Minimize saturated, *trans,* and polyunsaturated fats, and emphasize monounsaturated fats and fish oils or omega 3-fatty acids.

❖ Exercise is a must. Do it for your heart, breasts, mind, and soul. Exercise helps to control estrogen activity in the body, decreasing harmful estrogen and increasing healthy estrogen. Shoot for about five hours a week of some activity that you enjoy. Vary your exercise just as you vary your foods. To work different muscles, mix an aerobic-type, heartbeat-raising activity with something that stresses and strengthens the muscles.

❖ Calcium and magnesium help to build the bones and possibly lower blood pressure. Premenopausal women need 1,000 milligrams daily, and menopausal women require 1,500 milligrams. Your magnesium intake should be 500 to 650 milligrams per day (about half the dose of calcium). Take the two together in a combined supplement, and divide your doses into morning and nighttime supplements.

❖ Excessive salt, sugar, alcohol, caffeine, and soda pop have been reported to negatively affect bone density. Excessive alcohol (more than two glasses a day) is associated with an increased risk of breast cancer and osteoporosis. Minimize these in your diet.

❖ Drink about eight glasses of water each day. Water delivers nutrients to the cells, enables your glands and hormones to operate more efficiently, allows your liver to break down fat, releases excess water by causing you to urinate more, and keeps your skin and organs hydrated. Don't wait for nature to signal thirst; sip throughout the day.

❖ Get adequate sleep and rest. You will feel and look better. Our bodies and minds need time to repair and regenerate themselves. Avoid sedatives and pills, which artificially induce sleep. A warm glass of soy milk is helpful before bed, rather than a cup of coffee or tea (unless it's herb tea). The caffeine in tea and coffee tends to stimulate some people, making them restless and causing difficulties in falling asleep.

❖ Don't smoke. If you do, make a commitment to quit. Smoking increases the incidence of heart disease, hypertension, osteoporosis, lung cancer, and possibly breast cancer.

❖ Schedule regular check-ups with your doctor. Have your cholesterol levels tested, making sure you get the full panel and not just the total cholesterol count. If you haven't already done it, go in for a bone-density baseline test so that you and your doctor can monitor your bone health. If you are more than fifty years old (the age for breast screening has recently been reduced to forty in some countries), have a mammography screening at least every two years; some special situations call for yearly checks. And, of course, don't forget your annual Pap smear.

❖ Perform monthly breast self-examinations. The best time is following your period (if you are still having menstrual periods). If you don't have periods or if you've had a hysterectomy, pick a particular day of the month, such as the first or the last, and check yourself regularly on that day. If you find a lump, do not panic; make an appointment with your doctor to have it checked. Take along any old x-rays of the breast that you may have, or retrieve them from labs where they may be stored. The doctor and radiologist need to compare these to the new ones they'll take to determine if there have been any changes.

❖ Develop a positive attitude toward menopause and aging. Menopause is a natural phase of a woman's life. Some cultures look upon menopausal women with great respect and regard them as sources of wisdom. It is a time free from the fear of pregnancy and free from the chores of childbearing and child-rearing (for most women). It is new territory filled with different experiences and lessons. Prepare for it as much as you can, and learn to enjoy all that life has to offer.

## Not for Women Only

Although the natural estrogen diet is primarily aimed at perimenopausal and menopausal women, its health benefits extend to men, children, and other women. In men, added benefits include lowering the risk of prostate and bowel cancer. In premenopausal women, benefits include minimizing premenstrual symptoms and lowering the risk of breast and bowel cancer. In general, one or two servings of soy foods a day for men, children, and premenopausal women is adequate for cardiac and blood pressure benefits.

## Soy the Quick and Easy Way

Sometimes it's just hard to get a new program going. We are so driven by habit that trying foreign foods may be difficult, and the mere thought of altering our comfortable routines may be even more unappealing. This book helps you ease into the natural estrogen diet by offering suggestions that you can start tomorrow, without altering your usual routines too dramatically. After you've made small changes and gained courage, you can move on to some of the suggestions that you'd bypassed, or you might even experiment with some of the wonderful recipes found later in this book. The book also provides nutritional information for specific soy products, so you will be aware of the caloric content, fat, fiber, and calcium of these foods.

Below are some recommendations for integrating natural-estrogen foods into each of your daily meals.

*Snacks*

❖  Soy nuts
❖  Soy milk, flavored or plain
❖  Fresh green soybeans
❖  Soy yogurt
❖  Soy cheese on pita bread, tortillas, or crackers
❖  Smoothies made with soy protein or pureed tofu and your favorite fruits
❖  Oy-Soy Trail Mix (BodyLogic; see the Resources section)
❖  Rice Snackle Bars (BodyLogic)
❖  Cereal Crumble (BodyLogic)
❖  Trail mix (oats, rice, wheat, sunflower seeds)
❖  Carrots and cucumbers
❖  Apples, pears, grapes, and plums
❖  Papayas
❖  Crumble firm tofu in skillet and cook like scrambled eggs.
❖  Substitute soy flour (20 percent) in a muffin or pancake recipe.

## Breakfast

- ❖ Cereal Crumble (BodyLogic)
- ❖ Pour soy milk on high-fiber cereal.
- ❖ Mix soy yogurt into high-fiber cereal.
- ❖ Sprinkle flaxseed on high-fiber cereal.
- ❖ Sprinkle isolated soy protein (ISP) on cereal or fruit.
- ❖ Add ISP to baked goods.
- ❖ Blend two to four tablespoons of ISP into orange juice.
- ❖ Add prunes to high-fiber cereal, or eat plain.

## Lunch/Dinner

- ❖ Add fresh green soybeans to salads.
- ❖ Substitute soy milk for white sauce or pudding, or use as a base for cream soup.
- ❖ Use blended tofu as a base for cream soup.
- ❖ Cube firm tofu and add to soups, stews, casseroles, or chili.
- ❖ Eat takeout miso soup, or make it yourself (see recipe on page 94).
- ❖ Substitute creamed tofu for cheese in lasagna or enchiladas.
- ❖ Marinate firm tofu and grill, or make into kebobs.
- ❖ Grill tempeh like a burger.
- ❖ Add tofu or tempeh to vegetable soup.
- ❖ Stir-fry firm tofu with vegetables.
- ❖ Eat lentil or split-pea soup.
- ❖ Add carrots, beets, or cucumbers to salads.
- ❖ Put tofu chili on a baked potato.
- ❖ Make chili dogs from soy hot dogs and vegetarian chili; top with soy cheese.
- ❖ Add soy hot dogs to bean or pea soups.
- ❖ Make tofu tacos with crumbled firm tofu and taco spices.
- ❖ Buy or make soy burgers; put on wheat bun with lettuce, tomatoes, and onion.
- ❖ Make or buy low-fat coleslaw.

## Nutritional Content of Soy Foods

| | Soy Protein (grams) | Fat (grams) | Calories |
|---|---|---|---|
| miso (1 tablespoon) | 2 | 1 | 35 |
| soy flour (3½ ounces) | | | |
| regular | 35 | 22 | 441 |
| defatted | 47 | 1.2 | 329 |
| soy milk (1 cup) | | | |
| regular | 10 | 4 | 140 |
| reduced fat | 4 | 2 | 100 |
| soy nuts (1 ounce) | 13.3 | 5.5 | 127 |
| soy oil (1 tablespoon) | 0 | 13.6 | 120 |
| soy sprouts (½ cup) | 4.6 | 2.5 | 45 |
| soybeans, dried (½ cup, cooked) | 14.3 | 7.7 | 149 |
| soybeans, green, without pods (½ cup, cooked) | 6 | 2 | 60 |
| tofu (½ cup) | | | |
| firm | 13 | 6 | 120 |
| soft | 9 | 5 | 80 |
| silken | 9.6 | 2.4 | 72 |
| tempeh (½ cup) | 17 | 8 | 204 |
| TVP (1 cup, reconstituted) | 22 | 0.2 | 120 |

## Nutritional Content of Brand-Name Soy Drinks and Foods

| Drinks (1 cup unless indicated; each cup has approximately 300 milligrams of calcium) | Soy Protein (grams) | Fat (grams) | Calories |
|---|---|---|---|
| Edensoy Extra Original Soy Milk | 10 | 4 | 130 |
| Pacific Lite Plain | 4 | 2.5 | 100 |
| Pacific Lite Cocoa | 4 | 2 | 160 |
| Revival Soy Meal-Replacement Drink | 20 | 2.5 | 240 |
| Solair Vanilla Bean | 3 | 2 | 98 |
| Trader Joe's Soy-Um | 4 | 3 | 100 |
| VitaSoy Enriched Original | 6 | 3 | 110 |
| VitaSoy Enriched Vanilla | 6 | 3 | 140 |
| West Soy Dessert Drink (6 ounces) | 6 | 4 | 160 |
| **Foods** | | | |
| Boca Burger (original; 1) | 12 | 0 | 84 |
| BodyLogic Super Bumble Crumble (½ cup) | 14 | 15 | 310 |
| Fantastic Foods Mandarin Chow Mein with Tofu (1 package) | 22 | 5 | 330 |
| Hickory Baked Tofu (3 ounces) | 18 | 3.5 | 140 |
| Light Life Smart Dogs (1) | 9 | 0 | 45 |
| Morningstar Breakfast Links (2) | n/a | 5 | 90 |
| Nancy's Soy Yogurt (8 ounces) | 7 | 4 | 200 |
| Trader Joe's Eggless Salad (½ cup) | 7 | 8 | 120 |
| TofuRella Tofu Cheese (1 ounce) | 6 | 5 | 80 |
| Wildwood Tofu Cutlets (3 ounces) | 13 | 12 | 180 |
| Wildwood Veggie Burger (1) | 11 | 10 | 150 |
| Yamato Boiled Soybeans (½ cup) | 9 | 5 | 103 |
| Yves Veggie Cuisine Tofu Wieners (1) | 9 | 0 | 45 |

| Soy Powders | Soy Protein (grams) | Isoflavones (milligrams) |
| --- | --- | --- |
| Genisoy Natural Protein Powder (1 ounce) | 24 | 74 |
| Genisoy Soy Protein Shake (1 ounce) | 14 | 43 |
| Take Care Soy Protein Powder (1 ounce) | 20 | 57 |
| Twinlab Isoflavone Powder (1 teaspoon) | 34 | 85 |
| Whole Foods Soy Protein Powder (1 ounce) | 24 | 43 |

# PART II

✤

# Recipes

## Introduction

Telling someone to eat more soy is good advice. But showing you how to actually do it is another matter. In this chapter, we have compiled delicious, practical, and easy-to-prepare dishes incorporating soy products and other phytoestrogen-rich foods. Choose the recipes that you think you'll like, based on the ingredients that you already know, and then experiment with something new and exotic. After gaining confidence in phytoestrogen cooking, venture out and create your own dishes with the various soy products that are available in supermarkets. We hope you will be encouraged and inspired by your new cooking experiences.

The nutrient analysis for the original recipes in the Australian edition was calculated by Jenny Chan, a practicing consultant dietitian and nutritionist in Liverpool, New South Wales, Australia. Additional recipes from various contributors were arranged and annotated by Naomi Wise. Nutrient analysis of all recipes in this edition was calculated by Amy Demmon using the Nutritional Data Resources Nutrient Data Base. This analysis does not include optional variations. Equivalents for certain ingredients were supplied by Linda Ojeda.

People watching their weight can use low-fat soy milk and defatted soy flour in these recipes, although the latter can be difficult to find. Hopefully, defatted soy flour will become a common item in supermarkets and food stores in the future.

Those of you cooking for several people in a household can add chicken or other meat to the recipes so that the rest of your family won't miss out on their preferred protein. For example, in stir-fry dishes using tempeh or tofu cutlet, add some diced chicken for those who may not like these two ingredients. Lastly, those who are allergic to or intolerant of certain ingredients in the recipes should substitute or omit the offending ingredient from the recipe.

## Conversion Table

| Abbreviations: | g: grams | mL: milliliter | mm: millimeter |
| --- | --- | --- | --- |
| | kg: kilogram | L: liter | cm: centimeter |

| |
| --- |
| 1 teaspoon = 5 milliliters |
| 1 tablespoon = 3 teaspoons = 15 milliliters |
| 1 cup = 8 fluid ounces = 250 milliliters |
| 1 ounce = 30 grams |
| 1 gram = 0.035 ounce |
| 1 inch = 2.5 centimeters |
| 1 centimeter = 0.4 inch |
| 1 fluid ounce = 30 milliliters |
| 20 fluid ounces = 2½ cups = 625 milliliters |

# Glossary of Ingredients

Chickpeas (garbanzo beans)

Chili Sauce

Cooking oils

Garam Masala (Indian Spice
  Mixture)

Ketjap Manis

Low-Fat Ground Pork

Miso

Oyster Sauce

Soy Sauce, Light and Dark

Tahini

Tamarind

Tofu Buk (Deep-Fried Tofu)

Tofu Cutlets

### Chickpeas (garbanzo beans)

Chickpeas come cooked, in cans, or dried, in packages. They are very rich in phytoestrogens, proteins, and fiber. To cook dried chickpeas, see page 76.

### Chili Sauce

Chinese chili sauce is not the same as America's mild, tomatoey bottled chili sauce (for shrimp cocktails, etc.), nor is it a puree like some bottled Asian hot sauces. In Asian groceries and supermarkets with Asian food sections, look for bottled dark red sauce in which large quantities of chopped red hot peppers are visible. Vietnamese chili sauce is similar to Chinese. See p. 135 for a homemade version.

### Cooking oils

In the Asian recipes in this book, and for recipes requiring deep-frying, we have indicated a choice of soy oil, peanut oil, or canola oil. Soy oil contains phytoestrogens, but it is polyunsaturated and not always easy to find. Peanut oil is also unsaturated, but has the most authentic flavor for Asian dishes. If you are shopping for other ingredients at an Asian grocery, you can find Chinese peanut oils as well; the brand with the richest flavor is Lion and Globe. Canola oil is monounsaturated and the healthiest choice, but has no flavor of its own to contribute to foods; many people object to a "greasy" aftertaste. Olive oil, which is monounsaturated, has been specified wherever its distinctive flavor would make a positive contribution.

### Garam Masala (Indian Spice Mixture)

Garam masala is an aromatic Indian spice mixture (*masala*) that's much more widely used in India than curry powder. It's available from Indian food stores, some gourmet shops, and most spice catalogs. To make your own, see page 78.

### Ketjap Manis

Ketjap Manis is a sweet, thick soy sauce made in Indonesia. Its name is the basis of the English word "ketchup." It is available in Asian food stores, specialty food stores, and by mail order from specialty food catalogs.

### Low-Fat Ground Pork

Store-bought minced pork usually has a very high fat content (up to 30%). To decrease the fat content of the meat to that of skinless chicken breast, for each serving portion (of 3½ ounces), substitute 1 center-cut loin pork chop (about 4 ounces boneless or 5 ounces with bone). Remove visible fat, wash meat surface briefly under hot running water (this will remove bacteria), and, if you don't have a meat grinder, whir in a food processor or chop very fine with a knife. For a richer flavor (with somewhat higher fat), use a pork butt steak, trimming visible fat before processing, and picking over food-processed meat to remove any visible strings of unchopped gristle. (With small quantities as are used in this book, it should take just a minute.)

### Miso

There are 5 types of miso paste; the darker the color, the stronger and tangier the flavor. Some brands, such as Marukome, have dashi concentrate included, so there is no need to add dashi when you use them in soup. Please read the contents of the package carefully before making your purchase. Miso is also a tasty ingredient in salad dressings and in sauces for fish; for these purposes, choose miso without added dashi. Miso may be found in health food stores and Asian food stores, either on the shelves or in the refrigerated section. After opening, store in the refrigerator.

### Oils — *see* Cooking Oils

## Oyster Sauce

Oyster sauce is readily available from most supermarkets and Asian food stores. The sauce is made from extracts of oyster, caramel, and other additives. Brands do vary in content: Some contain MSG and preservatives, while others are preservative-free. Check the label before making your purchase. Once open, store in the refrigerator or, if the brand has preservatives and you expect to use the bottle quickly, you can store it in a cool cupboard.

## Pork, Ground — see Low-Fat Ground Pork

## Soy Sauce, Light and Dark

There are basically two types of Chinese soy sauce, light and dark. Other Asian countries mainly use light soy. The soy sauce brands most commonly available in North American supermarkets (Kikkoman, La Choy, etc.) are light soy sauces. At Asian groceries in the U.S. you can obtain not only dark soy, which is thick and glutinous because of its molasses content, but you can also find the more delicate-flavored light soys imported from China, Hong Kong, and Taiwan (brands such as Pearl River, Superior Soy, and Amoy). If there is no Asian market nearby, Tamari (a very rich Japanese soy sauce) is available at most health food stores and makes a passable substitute for dark soy. Add a generous pinch of sugar or a teaspoon of molasses to any recipe in which you are substituting a light soy or Tamari in place of dark soy.

## Tahini

A beige-colored bottled sauce made from ground or milled sesame seeds, tahini is available from health-food stores, Middle Eastern–style groceries and delis, and many super-markets. It is very rich in proteins, calcium, phosphorus, and vitamin E. Tahini also contains phytoestrogens. The oil in the tahini tends to separate from the solids, so stir thoroughly before using. Once opened, tahini should be refrigerated to prevent rancidity. Let it return to room temperature before use, as it is very hard to stir when cold.

## Tamarind

Tamarind is a tropical fruit with a tangy flavor. It is used in Asian and Hispanic cuisines. In Asian and Hispanic groceries it's usually sold as a packaged dried fruit or a dried concentrate. Rehydrate it in water and use as directed in cooking. East Indian food stores sell small bottles of thick liquid tamarind concentrate. The concentrate is convenient to use, but must be refrigerated after opening because in hot weather it may bubble over onto the cupboard shelf, even if the bottle is tightly capped.

## Tofu Buk (Deep-Fried Tofu)

Ready-fried tofu is sold in packages at Asian food stores. (If you cannot find it ready-made, see recipe, p. 79.) Fried tofu is light brown in color and rather spongy in texture.

## Tofu Cutlets

Tofu cutlets are compressed hard tofu that has been marinated in soy sauce or curry sauce and cooked again before packaging. You can often find tofu cutlets next to other tofu products in the refrigerated sections in supermarkets or health food stores. If unavailable, see recipes (p. 80).

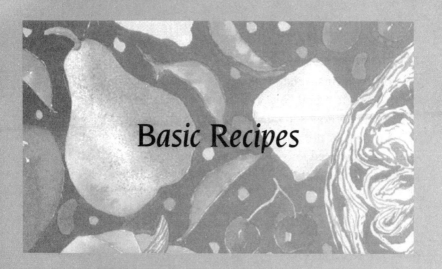

# Basic Recipes

Cooked Dried Chickpeas

Cooked Dried Soybeans

Asian-Style Chicken Stock

Garam Masala

Deep-Fried Tofu

Grilled or Broiled Tofu Cutlet

Plain Baked Tofu Cutlet

# COOKED DRIED CHICKPEAS

If using dried chickpeas, soak them overnight in cold water to cover. Drain, rinse, and place in a saucepan with ample water to cover. Bring to a boil, lower heat, and simmer for 1 to 2 hours, depending on how soft you like your chickpeas. The stock can be saved for use in other dishes, such as soups. Cooked chickpeas can be refrigerated for several days before use. A cup of dried chickpeas will expand to 2½-3 cups after soaking and cooking

# COOKED DRIED SOYBEANS

Soak soybeans overnight in cold water to cover. Rinse and discard any bad beans or debris. Drain off water. Place in a pressure cooker with 3¼ cups water. Bring to pressure and cook for 30 minutes. If cooking in an ordinary saucepan, cover with six to eight cups of water. Bring to a boil and simmer 2-3 hours on low heat, adding more water if liquid cooks away. Cooked soybeans may be refrigerated or frozen if desired. One cup of dried soybeans will expand to about 3 cups.

# ASIAN-STYLE CHICKEN STOCK

PER CUP: 38 CALORIES, 4.8 G PROTEIN, 1 G CARBOHYDRATE, 1.4 G FAT (.38 G SATURATED),
72 MG SODIUM, 0 G FIBER.

2 pounds bony chicken parts (backs, wing-tips, necks, feet if available)
2 qts. water for pressure cooking, or 2 qts. plus 2 cups for soup-pot cooking
2 slices fresh ginger
5 white peppercorns

Place chicken in a pressure cooker or in a large heavy pot with the water.

Add the ginger and peppercorns. In a pressure cooker, cook until pressurized, and then lower the heat to continue cooking for another 30 minutes. If cooking in a soup-pot, bring to a boil, skim grey foam from the top for five minutes, then lower heat and maintain at a lively simmer for two to three hours, until stock is richly flavored. If too much liquid cooks away, add a small amount of water and continue simmering.

Allow the stock to cool thoroughly, uncovered. (Covering it while it is hot will turn it sour.) Pour into a wide-mouthed bottle or similar covered container and refrigerate overnight or longer. Before using, skim all fat from the surface and discard it (or use it for other purposes).

Store in the refrigerator or freezer until ready to use. If you freeze the stock for use at a later date, it may be most convenient to divide it into portions suitable for use in recipes. This way, you'll only defrost the amount you need each time a recipe calls for stock. (Many cooks freeze chicken stock in an ice cube tray or in half-cup-sized custard cups. When the stock is frozen, they transfer these cubes or rounds into ziptop plastic bags for continued freezing.) Frozen stock keeps for about 14 weeks. Refrigerated stock keeps only 3 to 4 days.

**Note:** If you aren't using a pressure cooker, place the ingredients in a large soup-pot or saucepan and add an extra 2 cups water. Bring to a boil and simmer at least 2 hours before using.

Makes about 1 liter.

❖                                                                    ❖

Stock made from bony parts tends to have a higher calcium content. This can be increased by adding 1 tablespoon apple cider vinegar to the cooking pot. When beef stock is required, use 2 pounds meaty beef bones (shanks, shins) instead of chicken and, if cooking in a soup pot, simmer for 4 hours. Meaty pork bones can also be used to make stock using the above method. (Double the stovetop cooking time.) Any fat that you have not skimmed off will be very easy to remove once the stock has been chilled.

❖                                                                    ❖

# GARAM MASALA

PER TABLESPOON: 20 CALORIES, .8 G PROTEIN, 3.5 G CARBOHYDRATE,
.8 G FAT (0 G SATURATED), 1.9 MG SODIUM, 1 G FIBER.

2 tablespoons whole cardamom seeds
4 tablespoons ground cinnamon
2 tablespoons whole cloves
1 tablespoon whole cumin seeds
1 tablespoon mace
⅛ teaspoon ground nutmeg

Place all spices in a skillet and roast lightly over medium-high heat until the spices darken in color and smell fragrant. Grind together in a clean coffee grinder. Store in an airtight bottle away from heat and strong light.

*Recipe adapted from* Totally Hot *(Doubleday, 1986), by Michael Goodwin, Charles Perry, and Naomi Wise.*

# DEEP-FRIED TOFU

Cut firm tofu into 2-inch cubes or triangles of about 3 inches per side. Place on paper towels and let stand for several minutes to dry, then gently pat triangles on all sides with fresh paper towels. Heat a wok or large heavy skillet. Add 3-4 cups of cooking oil (soy, peanut, or canola) and bring oil to 375°F. One by one, slide the tofu triangles into the oil. If they stick together, gently separate them with long chopsticks or two long spoons. Fry until firm and golden all over, turning frequently. Remove with chopsticks or a slotted spoon and place on a double-thickness of paper towels. If you need to fry a second batch, be sure the oil has regained its temperature before beginning.

For later use, place fried tofu in a zip-top plastic bag or a covered container and refrigerate for up to five days. When cool, the oil may be strained into a bottle and refrigerated for future use in stir-fries.

# GRILLED OR BROILED
# TOFU CUTLET

firm tofu, sliced into slabs one inch thick
light soy sauce
dark (Asian) sesame oil

Place tofu on a paper towel to dry, then blot top with another paper towel. With a pastry brush, paint tofu with light soy sauce and then with sesame oil. If there is time, let marinate about an hour at room temperature.

Grill or broil tofu until well-browned. (It will survive the grill best if placed on a fine-mesh barbecue screen.) Turn it, paint again with soy and sesame, and continue cooking until browned and slightly crisp at the edges. If not using immediately, place in a covered container that will protect it from getting mashed, and refrigerate for up to five days.

Grilled tofu has a firm, chewy texture and a meaty flavor. Its flavors can be varied by marinating it in other mixtures, such as teriyaki sauce, Hoisin sauce, bottled Indian or Southeast Asian curry paste, or barbecue sauce (Western or Chinese).

# PLAIN BAKED TOFU CUTLET

Slice tofu into slabs about 1½ inch thick. Place on paper towels to dry, and blot the top with another paper towel. As tofu dries, preheat oven to 375°F. Place tofu on an ungreased baking pan and bake 20–30 minutes, until firm and dry. Pour off liquids from the pan. If not using immediately, store in a covered container, refrigerated, for up to 5 days.

Baked tofu is firm and chewy.

# Appetizers, Snacks, and Pick-Me-Ups

Chickpea Dip (Hummus)

Mutabbal (Baba Ghannouj)—
  Middle Eastern Eggplant Dip

Soybean Dip

Spicy Lentil Dip

Spring Rolls

Grilled Soy Cheese Sandwiches

Soy-Banana Breakfast Drink

Cantaloupe Soy Milk Shake

Strawberry Soy Drink

Tropical Fruit Smoothie

# CHICKPEA DIP (HUMMUS)

PER SERVING: 67 CALORIES, 2.6 G PROTEIN, 6.4 G CARBOHYDRATE, 3.5 G FAT (.5 G SATURATED), 251.4 MG SODIUM, 1.5 G FIBER.

1 cup cooked chickpeas (garbanzo beans)
3 cloves garlic, peeled
4 tablespoons tahini (see Glossary)
4 tablespoons boiling water
1 level teaspoon salt
¼ teaspoon ground black pepper
2 tablespoons plus 2 teaspoons lemon juice

Place all the ingredients in a blender or food processor, and blend until smooth. Add more lemon juice if desired. Serve as a dip with raw vegetables or savory crackers, or serve on top of baked potatoes.

**Note:** If using dried chickpeas, rinse with cold water and discard any bad chickpeas. Soak overnight in plenty of cold water. Drain and rinse chickpeas again. Place in a large saucepan, cover with cold water, and bring to a boil. Simmer for 30 minutes. Add ½ teaspoon salt halfway through the simmering time. About 3½ ounces of dried chickpeas will cook to 7 ounces in final weight.

Reduce the amount of garlic in this recipe if garlic on your breath worries you. Makes about 2 cups (10 servings) of dip.

❖                                                                    ❖

Chickpeas are quite sweet by themselves and have a very nice flavor. Most people can eat them unflavored. Roasted chickpeas are commonly eaten as a savory snack by young and old in Southeast Asian countries.

❖                                                                    ❖

# MUTABBAL (BABA GHANNOUJ) — MIDDLE EASTERN EGGPLANT DIP

PER SERVING: 155 CALORIES, 5.2 G PROTEIN, 11.6 G CARBOHYDRATE, 11.2 G FAT (1.71 G SATURATED), 346.9 MG SODIUM, 2.6 G FIBER.

2 large eggplants (about 2 pounds)
1 teaspoon salt
1 tablespoon chopped garlic
1 cup fresh-squeezed lemon juice
1 cup tahini
½ cup yogurt or soy yogurt

Preheat oven to 300°F. Place eggplants on a baking sheet and bake about 30 minutes, or until very soft and wrinkled. Remove from oven and allow to cool.

When you can handle the eggplants, remove their skins and place them in a colander in the sink to drain off the bitter brown liquid. Coarsely chop the eggplant flesh and place in a food processor or blender.

Place the salt on a cutting board and crush the garlic onto it with the side of a large knife (or squeeze through a garlic press). Add to the processor or blender. Add lemon juice and tahini, and puree thoroughly.

Turn mixture into a serving bowl and stir in the yogurt. Taste carefully and add more salt or lemon if desired. Serve with pita bread or wheat crackers.

*Recipe adapted from* Totally Hot (Doubleday, 1986), *by Michael Goodwin, Charles Perry, and Naomi Wise.*

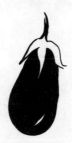

# SOYBEAN DIP

PER SERVING: 60 CALORIES, 3.4 G PROTEIN, 2.4 G CARBOHYDRATE, 4.4 G FAT (.6 G SATURATED), 209.9 MG SODIUM, .9 G FIBER.

2 teaspoons red or Italian onion, finely chopped
1 tablespoon plus 1 teaspoon olive or soybean oil
1 teaspoon curry powder
3 teaspoons water
¾ cup cooked soybeans (see p. 76)
¾ teaspoon salt
1 tablespoon plus 1 teaspoon boiling water
1 tablespoon plus 1 teaspoon light sour cream or unflavored low-fat yogurt

Place the onion and soybean oil in a small frying pan or skillet over medium heat. Mix the curry powder and water into a paste and add to the pan. Sauté for a few minutes, until fragrant but not dry.

Blend or process the curry mixture, soybeans, salt, boiling water, and sour cream until smooth. Serve as a dip with raw vegetables, water crackers, or other savory crackers as desired. This dip can be spread on bread and lightly toasted under the broiler (griller).

Makes just over 1 cup (7 servings) of dip.

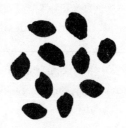

If you are using frozen cooked soybeans, rinse them in hot water before using in this recipe.

# SPICY LENTIL DIP

PER SERVING: 127 CALORIES, 8 G PROTEIN, 17.3 G CARBOHYDRATE, 3.4 G FAT (.8 G SATURATED), 139 MG SODIUM, 6.6 G FIBER.

1 cup lentils, rinsed and picked over
½ small onion, finely chopped
1 tablespoon plus 1 teaspoon olive or soybean oil
1 red chile, seeded and finely chopped
1 heaping teaspoon peeled fresh ginger, finely chopped
½ teaspoon ground cumin
¼ teaspoon ground turmeric
1½ cups chicken or beef stock (see page 77) or reduced-salt canned chicken broth
½ teaspoon garam masala (see p. 78)
½ teaspoon salt
2 tablespoons fine-shredded unsweetened coconut

Soak the lentils in cold water for an hour or two.

Place the onion and oil in a saucepan over medium heat. Sauté until the onion is translucent and starting to brown. Add the chile and ginger and continue to sauté, stirring, for 2 minutes. Add the cumin and turmeric and stir through well.

Drain the lentils and add to the mixture in the saucepan. Stir for 3 to 4 minutes before adding the broth. Reduce the heat to very low and simmer for 15 minutes.

Add the garam masala, salt, and coconut. Cook for a further 10 to 15 minutes. Remove from heat and let cool. Scrape into a food processor and blend for 2 minutes.

Serve cold with raw vegetables or savory crackers. This dip can also be served hot with steamed rice. Ready-made garam masala is available at East Indian groceries and by mail order.

Makes 1½ cups (8 servings) of dip.

Lentils are rich in fiber, proteins, iron, and potassium. This legume also contains phytoestrogens.

# SPRING ROLLS

PER SERVING: 307 CALORIES, 11.4 G PROTEIN, 28.4 G CARBOHYDRATE,
16.6 G FAT (3.7 G SATURATED), 1004.3 MG SODIUM, 3.6 G FIBER.

7 ounces ground pork (see Glossary and note below)
1 tablespoon plus 1 teaspoon light soy sauce
1 tablespoon plus 1 teaspoon oyster sauce
5 ounces bean sprouts or sprouts
¾ cup bamboo shoots
10 stalks garlic chives
frying oil
1 clove garlic, diced
5¾ cups cabbage, shredded
1¼ cups diced carrot
1 teaspoon salt
small pinch of ground black pepper
1 tablespoon plus 1 teaspoon cornstarch
scant ⅓ cup water
1 medium package spring-roll wrappers, 8-by-8-inch sheets

Marinate the pork in the light soy sauce and oyster sauce.

Rinse the bean sprouts. Cut the bamboo shoots into strips similar in size to the bean sprouts. Cut the chives into similar lengths. Drain well and pat dry with paper towels.

Heat 2 teaspoons oil in a wok over medium heat. Sauté the garlic in the oil until fragrant, and then add the pork and its marinade. Stir-fry for 3 minutes. Increase the heat to high before adding the cabbage, bamboo shoots, and carrots. Stir-fry for 2 minutes, and then add the bean sprouts, salt, pepper, and chives. Stir through well, then transfer to a metal colander to cool and drain off sauces.

Mix the cornstarch with the water to make a paste, and cook in the microwave on high for 45 seconds.

Divide the filling into 20 portions and wrap in the spring-roll wrappers, tucking in the ends of the wrapper as you roll. Seal the edges with the cornstarch paste. Heat cooking oil to deep-fry temperature (350°F) and deep fry the spring rolls a few at a time until well browned all over, then drain on a double thickness of paper towels. Allow cooking oil to regain heat between batches. (Alternatively, brush the wrappers with egg white, lay on a lightly greased cookie sheet, and bake in a preheated 325°F oven for 30 minutes.)

Serve hot with Chinese mustard, ketchup, plum sauce, or sweet and sour sauce.

Serves 6 to 10.

**Note:** Those who do not wish to use ground pork can substitute ground chicken in this recipe. Vegetarians can use deep-fried tofu (*tofu buk*); shred it into strips with a sharp knife before adding it to the recipe.

# GRILLED SOY CHEESE SANDWICHES

PER SERVING: 240 CALORIES, 13.7 G PROTEIN, 25.6 G CARBOHYDRATE,
10.5 G FAT (3.3 G SATURATED), 476 MG SODIUM, 2.5 G FIBER.

2 slices Crusty Soy Bread (p. 178) or whole grain bread
1 teaspoon butter or margarine
1 handful alfalfa sprouts plus extra for garnish
1 tablespoon plus 1 teaspoon shredded carrot
1 ounce soy cheese, grated
salt and freshly ground black pepper, to taste
cherry tomatoes, for garnish (optional)

Warm a sandwich grill or a waffle iron with the flat grill plates
in place.

Spread the bread thinly with butter or margarine. Grease 1
section of grill plate with the remaining butter.

Place 1 slice of bread, buttered side down, in the grill or waffle
iron. Pile on the alfalfa sprouts, carrot, and soy cheese. Season
with salt and pepper to taste.

Cover with the second slice of bread, this time buttered side
up. Close the lid of the sandwich grill or waffler and cook for 3 to
4 minutes.

Slice the sandwich in half diagonally. Serve garnished with the
extra alfalfa sprouts and cherry tomatoes (if using).

Serves 1.

Note: If you do not own a sandwich grill or waffle iron, toast the
bread lightly on one side under a hot broiler and then place the open
sandwiches back under the broiler until the soy cheese has melted.

❖                                                                    ❖

Alfalfa sprouts are a rich source of lignans, coumestans
(chemicals that have an estrogenic effect), and vitamin C. As fresh
sprouts are very lightweight, a package will last a few meals. A few
people dislike sprouts' green, beany taste, but this almost disappears when they're cooked inside a sandwich. Raw alfalfa sprouts
can garnish this and other sandwiches or be used in salads.

❖                                                                    ❖

# SOY-BANANA BREAKFAST DRINK

PER DRINK: 270 CALORIES, 5.4 G PROTEIN, 45.7 G CARBOHYDRATE,
8.9 G FAT (2.1 G SATURATED), 192.2 MG SODIUM, 1.8 G FIBER.

scant 1 cup soy milk
1 ripe banana, cut into small pieces
1 to 2 teaspoons sugar or artificial sweetener
3 to 4 drops vanilla extract (optional)

Pour the soy milk into a blender or food processor. Add the banana and sugar to taste, and vanilla extract, if using. Blend for 30 seconds. Chill before serving.

Makes 1 cup.

  Avoid bananas if you suffer from reflux problems or joint pains, as they may aggravate the condition.

# CANTALOUPE SOY MILK SHAKE

PER MILK SHAKE: 114 CALORIES, 6.1 G PROTEIN, 15.3 G CARBOHYDRATE,
3.5 G FAT (.4 G SATURATED), 39.7 MG SODIUM, .1.7 G FIBER.

8 ounces cantaloupe, peeled and diced
1 tablespoon plus 1 teaspoon rich dark honey
scant ½ cup fresh soy milk
7 ounces silken tofu

Place all the ingredients into a blender or food processor.
Blend for 1 minute. Chill before serving.
Makes about 3¼ cups.

❖ Cantaloupes are rich in beta-carotene, a compound linked to
lower lung cancer rates. The melons also have blood-thinning
properties, as they inhibit platelet aggregation and thus reduce the
risk of blood clots forming within blood vessels. ❖

# STRAWBERRY SOY DRINK

PER SERVING: 211 CALORIES, 4.9 G PROTEIN, 30 G CARBOHYDRATE, 8.7 G FAT (1.9 G SATURATED),
192.1 MG SODIUM, 2.6 G FIBER.

scant 1 cup soy milk
2 to 3 teaspoons sugar or artificial sweetener
¾ cup strawberries, washed, hulled, and sliced

Pour the soy milk into a blender or food processor.
Add the sugar or artificial sweetener to taste, and add the straw-
berries. Blend for 30 seconds. Chill before serving.
Makes 1 serving.

Commercially prepared soy milk is readily available. The UHT or long-life soy milk tastes different than homemade soy milk. Some preparations are fat-reduced, and these are particularly good for people on a weight-reduction diet. Some brands are calcium-enriched and therefore good for those who need more dietary calcium. Some brands of soy milk are already flavored and come in 8-fluid-ounce UHT packages, making them convenient for lunch or picnic packs.

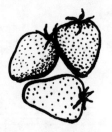

# TROPICAL FRUIT SMOOTHIE

PER SERVING: 222 CALORIES, 5 G PROTEIN, 33.2 G CARBOHYDRATE, 8.8 G FAT (2 G SATURATED), 192.1 MG SODIUM, 1.4 G FIBER.

½ cup fresh pineapple chunks
1 ripe banana
¼ teaspoons coconut extract
2 cups vanilla flavored soy milk*
4-6 ice cubes
pineapple wedge and toasted coconut for garnish

*Vitasoy Vanilla Delite or Light Vanilla or other brand

Blend all ingredients together in a blender until thick and smooth. Garnish with toasted coconut and pineapple wedge. Serves 2.

*Recipe from* Healthy and Delicious Recipes, Vol. 1. *By permission of Vitasoy.*

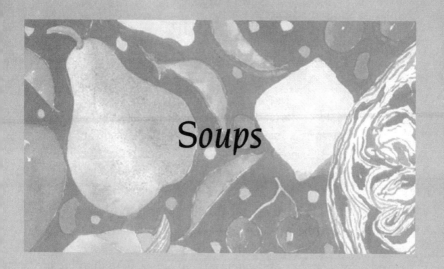

# Soups

Miso Soup

Creamy Corn Soup

Tomato Corn Chowder

Creamy Tomato Soup

Creamy Pumpkin Soup

Lentil-Vegetable Soup

Creamy Potato Soup

Curried Carrot Soup

# MISO SOUP

PER SERVING: 167 CALORIES, 14.4 G PROTEIN, 11.7 G CARBOHYDRATE,
8.1 G FAT (1.3 G SATURATED), 997.1 MG SODIUM, 3.8 G FIBER.

1 cup water
dashi stock paste (or concentrate, if using plain miso paste)
1 green onion, green part only, cut into ¾-inch lengths
3½ ounces tofu, cut into ½- to ¾-inch cubes
1 level tablespoon plus 1 level teaspoon miso paste (see Glossary)

Bring the water to a boil in a small saucepan. Add the dashi stock paste (if using) and allow to boil for 2 to 3 minutes. Add the green onion and tofu.

Add a small amount of water to the miso paste to dissolve it evenly before adding to soup. Bring to a boil and serve in a deep bowl.

Serves 1.

**Note:** Firm tofu is normally used in this recipe, but many people prefer the soup with smooth, tender silken tofu instead.

❖ Miso soup is a popular Japanese breakfast dish for women and men. Dashi paste is available from Asian food stores and the Asian food sections of large supermarkets. ❖

# CREAMY CORN SOUP

PER SERVING: 226 CALORIES, 19.3 G PROTEIN, 27.8 G CARBOHYDRATE,
5.5 G FAT (1 G SATURATED), 1337.8 MG SODIUM, 1.2 G FIBER.

2 tablespoons plus 2 teaspoons cornstarch
1 tablespoon plus 1 teaspoon light soy sauce
2 ounces skinless, boneless chicken breast meat, cut into thin strips
4 cups chicken stock (p. 77) or canned chicken broth
1 can creamed corn
5 ounces silken tofu
¼ cup water
1 large egg, beaten
salt, to taste

Blend 2 teaspoons of the cornstarch with the soy sauce. Add the chicken strips and allow to marinate for at least 10 minutes.

Bring the chicken stock to a boil in a large saucepan. Add the marinated chicken, lower the heat, and simmer for 5 minutes. Stir in creamed corn.

Whirl tofu and water in a blender or food processor for 1 minute. Add the blended tofu and the egg to the soup mixture, stirring constantly.

If you prefer a thicker, glossier soup, mix the remaining cornstarch into a paste using a little water, and then use it to thicken the soup. Add salt according to taste or dietary restrictions. Serve hot.

Serves 4 to 6.

❖   This is a very creamy and tasty recipe. Omit the tofu if   ❖
you do not enjoy a creamy taste. Add extra cornstarch if a thicker
soup is desired. A very tasty variation of this soup substitutes crab
meat for chicken. (Add the crab meat just a minute before adding
the tofu.) In West Africa, a spicy version is popular: Substitute
chopped raw shrimp or prawns for the chicken, and stir in cayenne
or hot sauce until soup is quite spicy to your taste. The African version can be made with water instead of stock for pisceo-vegetarians.
Both the corn and tofu in this recipe contain phytoestrogens. Omit
the egg if you are on a low-cholesterol diet.

# TOMATO CORN CHOWDER

PER SERVING: 329 CALORIES, 8.3 G PROTEIN, 53.1 G CARBOHYDRATE,
11.4 G FAT (1.8 G SATURATED), 871.8 MG SODIUM, 6.9 G FIBER.

1 onion diced
1 tablespoon vegetable oil
2 carrots, cut in half lengthwise and sliced
2 stalks celery, thinly sliced
1–2 cloves garlic, mashed
2 cups water, or vegetable stock
2 medium sized potatoes, peeled and diced
¾ to 1 cup corn, fresh or frozen kernels
2 tablespoons soy sauce
1 teaspoon basil, dried; 1 tablespoon fresh minced basil
1 bay leaf
2 Roma tomatoes, peeled, seeded, and diced
2 cups soy milk*
Salt to taste
¼ teaspoon black pepper, or to taste
pinch of cayenne, or to taste
grated Parmesan cheese, to taste

*Vitasoy or other brand

Heat oil in a 2-quart saucepan until fragrant. Add onions and
sauté until translucent. Add carrots, celery, and garlic and sauté 2-
3 minutes.

Add water or stock, potatoes, corn, and other seasonings.
Bring to a simmer and cook for about 15 minutes, until potatoes
are soft.

Add tomatoes and soy milk, and bring to a slow simmer.
Adjust seasonings, salt, and pepper. Serve with a sprinkle of
Parmesan cheese on top.

*Recipe from* Healthy and Delicious Recipes, Vol. 1. *By permission of*
*Vitasoy.*

# CREAMY TOMATO SOUP

PER SERVING: 339 CALORIES, 20.1 G PROTEIN, 26.1 G CARBOHYDRATE,
19.4 G FAT (1.3 G SATURATED), 393.9 MG SODIUM, 1.5 G FIBER.

2 teaspoons cooking oil
1 medium onion, diced
1 large tomato, diced
½ teaspoon chopped garlic
1 teaspoon fresh basil, chopped
½ teaspoon salt
½ teaspoon white pepper
1 cup soy milk
1 10½-ounce package firm silken tofu

Heat oil until fragrant in a saucepan. Add onion and sauté for 3 minutes or until transparent. Add tomato and garlic and continue to sauté for 2-3 minutes. Add basil, salt, and pepper. Blend in soy milk. Cook over medium-high heat, stirring constantly for 1 minute. Remove from heat and cool briefly.

Transfer to a food processor, add tofu, and puree until smooth. Serve hot or chilled.

Serves 3-4.

*Recipe courtesy of the Indiana Soybean Board.*

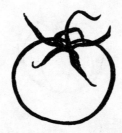

# CREAMY PUMPKIN SOUP

PER SERVING: 205 CALORIES, 6.3 G PROTEIN, 36.9 G CARBOHYDRATE,
4.5 G FAT (1.2 G SATURATED), 483.7 MG SODIUM, 7.3 G FIBER.

1 pound pumpkin, diced
1 medium apple, peeled and diced
1 medium potato, peeled and diced
1 medium onion, peeled and diced
1⅔ cups chicken stock (p. 77) or one 14-ounce can chicken stock or vegetable
broth plus 2 teaspoons extra
1⅔ cups soy milk
1 tablespoon plus 1 teaspoon cornstarch
salt and freshly ground black pepper, to taste
sprigs of fresh parsley, to garnish

Place the pumpkin, apple, potatoes, and onions into a large saucepan. Add the broth.

Bring to a boil and simmer for 20 minutes.

Blend or process the soup mixture until smooth, and then return it to the pan. Add the soy milk and bring to a boil once more.

If you prefer a thicker, glossier soup, mix the cornstarch with 2 teaspoons water and add to the soup. Allow to thicken slightly, then add salt and pepper to taste. Garnish with the parsley (if desired) and serve hot.

Serves 4 to 6.

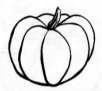

❖    The pumpkin, apple, and potato in this recipe all contain
phytoestrogens. If a creamier soup is desired, replace the soy milk
with 5 ounces silken tofu blended into a smooth purée with 1⅔
cups water or broth.    ❖

# LENTIL-VEGETABLE SOUP

PER SERVING: 272 CALORIES, 16.9 G PROTEIN, 49 G CARBOHYDRATE, 2 G FAT (.7 G SATURATED),
1585.7 MG SODIUM, 12.7 G FIBER.

½ cup red lentils, rinsed and picked over
¼ cup white pearl barley, rinsed and picked over
8 cups chicken stock (p. 77) or canned chicken broth or vegetable broth
2 large potatoes, diced
1 carrot, diced
3 tomatoes, diced
1 onion, diced
sprigs of fresh parsley, to garnish (optional)

Bring the lentils, pearl barley, and stock to a boil in a large
saucepan. Allow to simmer for 1 hour.

Add the potatoes, carrot, tomatoes, and onion to the soup
mixture. Simmer for a further 40 minutes.

Serve hot, garnished with the parsley (if using).

Serves 4 to 6.

**Note:** Instead of soup stock, you can use 2 pounds pork bones or
chicken bones; remove the bones before adding the vegetables.

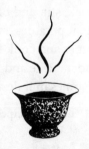

> ❖  Celery can substitute for onions and tomatoes. Packaged
> soup mixes containing pearl barley, split peas, lentils, and so on
> can be used instead of lentils and pearl barley. The red lentils, pearl
> barley, carrots, and potatoes in this recipe all contain
> phytoestrogens.

# CREAMY POTATO SOUP

PER SERVING: 389 CALORIES, 9.2 G PROTEIN, 49.4 G CARBOHYDRATE,
18.1 G FAT (2.6 G SATURATED), 1067.7 MG SODIUM, 5.1 G FIBER.

3 tablespoons vegetable oil
1 onion, diced
2–3 carrots, peeled and diced
2 medium-sized potatoes, peeled and diced
1 tablespoon dried dill
¼ teaspoon ground white pepper
2 teaspoons minced garlic
4 cups vegetable stock
2¼ cups soy milk*
1 cup instant mashed potatoes
salt and freshly ground white pepper to taste
grated Parmesan (optional)

*Vitasoy Creamy Original or other brand

In a heavy saucepan, 3-quart-capacity or larger, heat oil until fragrant. Gently sauté onions, carrots, and potatoes until onions are translucent. Add dill, white pepper, and garlic, and continue to sauté 2-3 minutes. Add stock, stir, and bring to a light simmer.

Add soy milk and instant potatoes, stirring thoroughly to blend. Bring to a light simmer and cook for about 12-15 minutes until potatoes are firm-tender. Taste and adjust seasonings. Sprinkle top with grated Parmesan if desired.

*Recipe from* Healthy and Delicious Recipes, Vol. 1. *By permission of Vitasoy.*

# CURRIED CARROT SOUP

PER SERVING: 85 CALORIES, 3.4 G PROTEIN, 15.2 G CARBOHYDRATE, 1.7 G FAT (.4 G SATURATED), 453.8 MG SODIUM, 3.9 G FIBER.

6 medium carrots
2 cups vegetable stock
1 small onion, chopped
2 teaspoons curry powder
½ cup plain soy milk

Combine all ingredients except the soy milk and cook over medium heat until carrots are tender. Pour into a blender and puree until smooth. Stir in the soy milk. Cook over low heat until hot.
Serves 4.

*Recipe courtesy of the Indiana Soybean Board.*

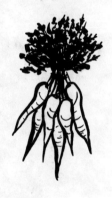

# Salads, Dressings, and Side Dishes

Chickpea Salad

Bean Salad

Thai Salad

Apple and Potato Salad

Soy Macaroni Salad

Greek Tofu Salad

Green Soybean Salad

Summertime Pickled Curried
  Vegetables

Tofu Mayonnaise

Creamy Poppy Seed Dressing

Healthy Caesar Salad Dressing

Creamy Basil Dressing

Curried Chickpeas

Spicy Chickpeas

Stir-Fried Green Beans
  with Pine Nuts

Stir-Fried Prawns, Snow Peas,
  and Tofu

Bean Sprouts in Fish Sauce

Cheesy Scalloped Potatoes

Fried Rice

# CHICKPEA SALAD

PER SERVING: 186 CALORIES, 7 G PROTEIN, 23.2 G CARBOHYDRATE, 6.7 G FAT (.6 G SATURATED), 679.7 MG SODIUM, 5.5 G FIBER.

1½ cups cooked or canned chickpeas (garbanzo beans), rinsed well and drained (see Glossary)
1 large or 2 medium ripe tomatoes, diced
½ cup diced celery
6 stalks fresh chives, finely chopped
2 sweet basil leaves, finely chopped

### Dressing:
2 cloves garlic, diced
1 tablespoon plus 1 teaspoon olive or canola oil
¼ teaspoon ground black pepper
¼ teaspoon ground cinnamon
½ teaspoon salt, or to taste
1 teaspoon sugar
1 tablespoon plus 1 teaspoon lemon juice
1 tablespoon plus 1 teaspoon light soy sauce

Make the dressing first. Sauté the garlic in the oil until golden brown. Discard garlic and set the oil aside until cool.

Place the garlic oil, pepper, cinnamon, salt, sugar, lemon juice, and soy sauce in a glass jar or bottle with a lid. Seal the jar and shake the ingredients together. Taste for seasoning and correct if necessary. Set aside.

Toss the chickpeas, tomatoes, and celery in a salad bowl. Shake the dressing once more and pour over the salad. Toss in the chives and sweet basil.

Serve with roasted chicken or barbecue, or as part of a vegetarian salad assortment.

Serves 4 to 6.

# BEAN SALAD

PER SERVING: 249 CALORIES, 9.9 G PROTEIN, 16.3 G CARBOHYDRATE,
17.4 G FAT (2.6 G SATURATED), 390.4 MG SODIUM, 3.7 G FIBER.

1 14-ounce can or jar three-bean mix, about 8 ounces drained
1 cup cooked soybeans
1 cup green (string) beans, ends trimmed
2 teaspoons red pepper, seeded and diced
2 teaspoons onions, finely diced
½ teaspoon salt
¼ teaspoon ground cinnamon
¼ teaspoon ground nutmeg
¼ teaspoon ground black pepper
3 tablespoons olive oil
1 tablespoon wine vinegar
2 teaspoons sugar, or to taste

Drain the three-bean mix and wash with cool boiled water, and then stir in the cooked soybeans.

Blanch the green beans in some salted, boiling water for 2 to 3 minutes, depending on thickness, until crisp-tender. Quickly refresh in cold water, drain, and cut into ¾-inch lengths. Add to the bean mixture.

Mix the remaining ingredients together. Taste for seasoning, and correct if necessary. Toss with the beans. Store in the refrigerator until ready to use, tossing a few times just before serving to mix the salad thoroughly with the dressing.

Serve cold at picnics, barbecues, or with vegetarian dinner platters.

Serves 4 to 6.

**Note:** If you are a diabetic, substitute artificial sweetener for the sugar.

# THAI SALAD

PER SERVING: 259 CALORIES, 18.5 G PROTEIN, 13.8 G CARBOHYDRATE,
16.4 G FAT (1.4 G SATURATED), 253.1 MG SODIUM, 3.3 G FIBER.

## Dressing:

1 tablespoon plus 1 teaspoon chopped fresh coriander
(Chinese parsley, cilantro) leaves
1 clove garlic, finely diced
2 tablespoons plus 2 teaspoons lime juice
1 tablespoon plus 1 teaspoon rice wine (or apple cider) vinegar
4 tablespoons nam pla (Thai fish sauce; see note)
1 small fresh hot red chile, diced
2 tablespoons plus 2 teaspoons boiling water
3 teaspoons sugar
½ teaspoon salt
2 teaspoons olive, peanut, or canola oil

## Thai Salad:

5 ounces lettuce, rinsed and drained
½ cup cucumber
⅓ cup red bell pepper
2 ounces fresh bean sprouts, rinsed and drained
3½ ounces fried tofu cubes (tofu buk) (see Deep-Fried Tofu, p. 79)
6 cherry tomatoes, rinsed and drained
fresh coriander (Chinese parsley, cilantro) leaves, to garnish
2 tablespoons plus 2 teaspoons shelled roasted peanuts, to garnish

Blend all the ingredients for the dressing in a food processor.
Set aside in the refrigerator until ready to use. This quantity makes
about ⅔ cup dressing.

To make the salad, tear the lettuce into small, bite-size portions. Cut the cucumber into chunks (skin may be left on if it has
no wax coating), shred the bell pepper, and remove the stringy
tails from the bean sprouts. Cut the fried tofu cubes into quarters
and slice the cherry tomatoes into halves if desired.

Arrange the salad vegetables in a dish or platter, and garnish with the fresh coriander leaves.

Crush the roasted peanuts and sprinkle on top of the salad just before serving. Pour the dressing over the salad and serve immediately.

Serves 4.

**Note:** Fish sauce can be found in the Asian-food sections of most grocery stores. This is an important ingredient for the dressing and gives the salad a unique taste.

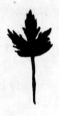

# APPLE AND POTATO SALAD

PER SERVING: 149 CALORIES, 4.8 G PROTEIN, 22.6 G CARBOHYDRATE, 4.9 G FAT (1 G SATURATED), 641.7 MG SODIUM, 2.3 G FIBER.

1 pound small or new potatoes
1 large green apple
1 tablespoon plus 1 teaspoon lime juice
¾ ounce lean packaged ham, diced (optional), or any soy-based smoked "meat"
4 to 5 stalks fresh chives, snipped
½ cup celery, fairly thinly sliced
6 tablespoons plus 2 teaspoons mayonnaise (low-fat or tofu; see page 114)
1 level teaspoon salt
freshly ground black pepper

Scrub the potatoes, removing any eyes or dirt. Do not peel. Place in a saucepan half-filled with water, bring to a boil, and cook for 12 minutes. Drain and allow to cool.

Wash and core the apple, but do not remove the skin. Cut into ½- to ¾-inch cubes and immediately mix with the lime juice. This process is called acidulation and helps prevent the apple from discoloring. Refrigerate until ready to use.

Cool the potatoes and cut into ½- to ¾-inch chunks. Mix the ham with the potatoes. Add the chives and celery. Mix in the mayonnaise, salt, a few grindings of pepper, and the acidulated apples. Let marinate in the refrigerator for an hour or so before serving.

Serves 6 to 8.

**Note:** Diced cooked chicken breast can be used instead of ham in this recipe. Vegetarians may substitute the above with nuts such as walnuts or pistachios, or use sunflower seeds

Apples contain estrone, which is a natural estrogen that circulates in the blood of postmenopausal women. Other foods such as rice also contain estrone, as well as estradiol. **Estradiol** predominantly circulates in the blood of premenopausal women. Pomegranates contain estrone, too; hence their Chinese nickname, the "fertility fruit."

# SOY MACARONI SALAD

PER SERVING: 192 CALORIES, 6.1 G PROTEIN, 26.6 G CARBOHYDRATE,
6.9 G FAT (1.1 G SATURATED), 418.6 MG SODIUM, 2.4 G FIBER.

7 ounces soy macaroni
1 cup frozen green peas
¾ ounce lean packaged ham, diced
2 teaspoons onion, diced
¼ level cup shredded carrot
¼ teaspoon salt
¼ teaspoon sugar
freshly ground black pepper, to taste
½ cup light mayonnaise or tofu mayonnaise (see page 114)
1 tablespoon grated cheese (optional)

Cook the soy pasta in 6 cups boiling salted water for 12 minutes. Cool quickly in cold water and drain well.

Cook the peas in boiling water for 2 or 3 minutes, until tender. Cool quickly in cold water and drain well.

Combine all the ingredients except the cheese and refrigerate for at least 1 hour before serving.

Add your favorite shredded cheese if you desire a cheesy flavor, and serve cold at picnics or barbecues. A green salad complements this dish very nicely.

Serves 4 to 6.

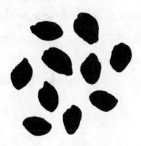

# GREEK TOFU SALAD

PER SERVING: 137 CALORIES, 8.7 G PROTEIN, 5.6 G CARBOHYDRATE,
9.9 G FAT (1.4 G SATURATED), 106.8 MG SODIUM, 1.9 G FIBER.

14 ounces extra-firm tofu,* drained and cut into ½-inch cubes
½ ounce sun-dried tomatoes (not oil packed)
1 tablespoon soaking water from sun-dried tomatoes
1½ teaspoons dried oregano
1 tablespoon olive oil
1 tablespoon red wine vinegar
12 pitted Kalamata olives, each cut into 3 pieces
1 tablespoon chopped red onion
⅔ cup ½-inch diced English cucumber
1 tablespoon chopped parsley
Salt and pepper to taste
butter lettuce for garnish

*Azumaya or other brand

Barely cover tomatoes with hot water in small bowl; let stand
20 minutes. Drain and reserve soaking water. Chop tomatoes.

Mix 1 tablespoon soaking water, oregano, olive oil, red wine
vinegar, sun-dried tomatoes, olives, and onion in a serving bowl.
Add tofu and gently toss to mix. Let stand 1 to 2 hours for flavors
to blend.

Just before serving, scatter with cucumber, parsley, salt, and
pepper. Mix lightly. Line each salad plate with butter lettuce leaf.
Mound tofu salad onto lettuce.

Serves 4.

*Recipe from* Delicious and Easy Recipes for Tofu and Pasta. *By permission
of Azumaya.*

# GREEN SOYBEAN SALAD

PER SERVING: 184 CALORIES, 15.4 G PROTEIN, 4.4 G CARBOHYDRATE,
8.9 G FAT (1.3 G SATURATED), 112 MG SODIUM, 4.9 G FIBER.

2 cups fresh green soybeans
½ cup finely chopped celery
¼ cup chopped green pepper
1 large tomato, diced
⅓ cup salad dressing of choice (such as low-fat French dressing)
Lettuce

In a large bowl, combine the soybeans, celery, green pepper, tomato, and dressing. Toss. Serve the salad on a bed of lettuce. Yields 4 servings.

*Recipe courtesy of the Indiana Soybean Board.*

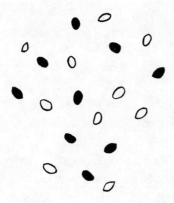

# SUMMERTIME PICKLED CURRIED VEGETABLES

PER SERVING: 467 CALORIES, 14.8 G PROTEIN, 26.3 G CARBOHYDRATE,
37.5 G FAT (4.5 G SATURATED), 1638 MG SODIUM, 8.4 G FIBER.

This vegetarian dish will delight your taste buds with sweet, sour, savory, hot, and spicy flavors, and it offers a varied texture to accompany your main meal or barbecues.

This dish is prepared a few days ahead of time and stored in the refrigerator until ready to use. The sauce needs a few days to infuse into the vegetables and "pickle" them. This dish is always served cold.

1¾ cucumber
3 long red chiles (such as fresh chile Numex, Italian frying peppers, or ripe Anaheims)
1 cup carrots
½ cup green (string) beans
5¾ cups cabbage
4 cups cauliflower
2 tablespoons plus 2 teaspoons sesame seeds
8 cloves garlic
1 medium onion
2 tablespoons plus 2 teaspoons curry powder
¼ cup water
6 tablespoons plus 2 teaspoons cooking oil (soy, peanut, canola)
¾ cup apple cider vinegar
2 tablespoons plus 2 teaspoons sugar
2 tablespoons plus 2 teaspoons salt
¼ teaspoon monosodium glutamate (MSG) (optional; see note)
¼ cup crushed roasted peanuts

Rinse all the vegetables and cut the cucumber, chiles, and carrots into strips. Slice the beans into 1¾-inch lengths and the cabbage into ¾ × 2-inch pieces. Cut the cauliflower into florets.

Spread all the vegetables out on baking trays or sheets. Place out in the sun for at least 4 hours to semi-dry the vegetables.

Lightly toast the sesame seeds in a frying pan or skillet, and set aside. Bruise the garlic and cut into quarters. Dice the onion very finely.

Make the curry powder into a paste with the water.

Heat the oil in a hot wok. Sauté the onion for a minute, and then add the curry paste and reduce the heat to medium. Sauté until the mixture is very fragrant before adding the vinegar, sugar, salt, and, if desired, MSG.

Increase the heat to high once more, and add the carrots, cabbage, and cauliflower. Mix well before adding the beans and garlic. Make sure the sauce is boiling before adding the chile and cucumber. Stir quickly and, when the sauce has returned to a boil, transfer to a shallow dish and allow to cool.

Sprinkle the peanuts and sesame seeds over the top. Serve cold. This spicy relish is good with satay or teriyaki chicken, or in fact with any barbecue or picnic foods

Serves 8 to 12.

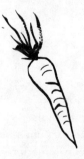

**Note:** The best results are achieved when this dish is cooked a day or two ahead of time. It will keep for up to a week in the refrigerator. Some people are extremely sensitive to monosodium glutamate, a flavoring often used in Asian cooking. Omit this entirely if you are sensitive to or dislike this ingredient.

The vegetables listed above are those commonly used in this dish. However, if one of the vegetables is out of season, you can simply omit it from the recipe.

# TOFU MAYONNAISE

PER TABLESPOON: 134 CALORIES, 5.1 G PROTEIN, 2.5 G CARBOHYDRATE,
11.4 G FAT (1.3 G SATURATED), 501.9 MG SODIUM, .1 G FIBER.

5 ounces tofu, preferably silken tofu
1 tablespoon plus 1 teaspoon boiling water
2 stalks fresh chives
2½ teaspoons white vinegar
1 tablespoon plus 1 teaspoon olive oil
1 teaspoon sugar or to taste
½ teaspoon salt or to taste
½ teaspoon English or other hot mustard

Place all the ingredients in a blender or food processor. Blend
for 30 seconds. Scrape down the sides of the blender, and blend
again until a smooth consistency is achieved. Taste and adjust
sugar and salt. Stir in additions.

Transfer the mayonnaise to a clean, airtight container and
store in the refrigerator until ready to use.

Makes about ¾ cup.

❖            Lemon or lime juice can be used in place of the vinegar in
this recipe, but vinegar has some preservative properties. Hence,
your mayonnaise will keep for a few days longer if made with vinegar rather than lemon or lime juice. Silken tofu is best for this
recipe, and it must be fresh. Vacuum-sealed packs are more likely
to be superior.

# CREAMY POPPY SEED DRESSING

PER TABLESPOON: 80 CALORIES, 1.2 G PROTEIN, 4.4 G CARBOHYDRATE,
6.3 G FAT (.1 G SATURATED), 121.7 MG SODIUM, .2 G FIBER.

1 cup soy oil
4 ounces soft silken tofu
½ cup honey
½ cup white vinegar
2 tablespoons poppy seeds
1½ teaspoons dry mustard
1¼ teaspoons salt
1 teaspoon paprika
2 tablespoons minced onion

Blend all ingredients except onions together in food processor until smooth and creamy. Stir in onions and mix well.

Makes 2½ cups.

*Recipe from* It's Soy Easy…to Cook with Soy. *By permission of the Ohio Soybean Council.*

# HEALTHY CAESAR
# SALAD DRESSING

PER TABLESPOON: 93 CALORIES, 3.1 G PROTEIN, .4 G CARBOHYDRATE,
8.1 G FAT (0 G SATURATED), 13.7 MG SODIUM, .1 G FIBER.

½ cup soy oil
1 teaspoon minced garlic
4 ounces soft silken tofu
1 tablespoon white wine vinegar
1 tablespoon lemon juice
2 teaspoons Dijon mustard
1 teaspoon lemon pepper
⅛ teaspoon Worchestershire sauce

In food processor or blender, combine all ingredients and
blend until smooth. Makes 1 cup. Toss with romaine lettuce and
croutons.

*Recipe from* It's Soy Easy…to Cook with Soy. *By permission of the Ohio
Soybean Council.*

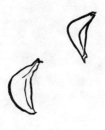

# CREAMY BASIL DRESSING

PER TABLESPOON: 37 CALORIES, .7 G PROTEIN, 2.1 G CARBOHYDRATE,
2.9 G FAT (.54 G SATURATED), 29.9 MG SODIUM, 0 G FIBER.

2 cups soy milk*
juice of 1 lemon
1 clove of garlic
6 fresh basil leaves
1 tablespoon olive oil
1 tablespoon vegetable oil
½ teaspoon dill weed
¼ teaspoon black pepper
dash of cayenne pepper
dash of salt
1 tablespoon grated Parmesan cheese

*Vitasoy Creamy Original or other brand

Whirl first four ingredients together in a processor or blender, slowly dribbling in oils through the opening while processing. Add remaining ingredients and blend briefly.

Makes about 2 cups.

*Recipe from* Healthy & Delicious Recipes, Vol. 1. *By permission of Vitasoy.*

# CURRIED CHICKPEAS

PER SERVING: 172 CALORIES, 4.3 G PROTEIN, 15 G CARBOHYDRATE,
10.2 G FAT (1.9 G SATURATED), 684.2 MG SODIUM, 3.4 G FIBER.

7 ounces dried chickpeas (garbanzo beans) or 1 13- to 16-ounce can of chickpeas

pinch of baking soda

3½ ounces dried tamarind or tamarind paste (or 1 tablespoon bottled tamarind
concentrate from India)

1¾ cups water

2 tablespoons plus 2 teaspoons cooking oil

1 medium onion, peeled and chopped

1¾-inch piece of fresh ginger, peeled and finely grated

4 green chiles, chopped and seeded

1 teaspoon salt

¼ teaspoon cayenne

1½ teaspoons garam masala (see p. 78)

2 lemons, thinly sliced, to garnish

½ cup coriander (Chinese parsley, cilantro) leaves, chopped, to garnish

Rinse the dried chickpeas, discarding any bad ones. Soak the
chickpeas overnight in cold water with the baking soda.

Soak the dry tamarind or tamarind paste in a scant ½ cup of
water. Remove the seeds and pulp, and strain and reserve the juice
for cooking.

If using dry chickpeas, pressure-cook in 1¼ cups water for 10
minutes (see the box below). Depressurize carefully and drain the
chickpeas. Reserve the cooking water. If using canned chickpeas,
drain them and reserve the can liquid.

Heat the oil in a deep frying pan or skillet. Add the onion and
ginger and sauté until brown, and then add the green chiles, salt,
cayenne, garam masala, and drained chickpeas. Sauté for a few
minutes. Stir in the reserved tamarind juice and the cooking water
from the pressure cooker or the can. (If using tamarind concentrate, stir thoroughly to dissolve it with the other ingredients.)

Simmer until the gravy becomes quite thick. Remove from the heat and transfer to a deep serving dish. Garnish with the lemon and coriander, and serve hot with steamed rice, pappadams, or chapatis.

Serves 4 to 6.

*Recipe adapted from an original by Dr. A. Gulati.*

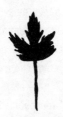

❖ Chickpeas contain second-class proteins and phytoestrogens. They are conveniently available cooked in cans, as well as in dried form. ❖

The chickpeas can be cooked in a heavy-based saucepan for 1 hour if you do not have a pressure cooker, although the latter reduces cooking time significantly. If you own a pressure cooker, take advantage of it by using it for fast cooking of legumes.

Dried tamarind is available in Hispanic and Asian groceries, and tamarind concentrate can be found in East Indian groceries. (Keep the latter refrigerated after opening.) You can substitute apple cider vinegar for tamarind in this recipe. Ready-made garam masala is available in East Indian groceries and is readily available by mail from spice catalogs. (See p. 78 to make at home.) ❖

# SPICY CHICKPEAS

PER SERVING: 135 CALORIES, 4.6 G PROTEIN, 15.7 G CARBOHYDRATE,
5.8 G FAT (.8 G SATURATED), 633.4 MG SODIUM, 4 G FIBER.

7 ounces chickpeas (garbanzo beans), or 1 13- to 16-ounce can of chickpeas
1¾ cups plus 1 tablespoon water to cook dried chickpeas
1 tablespoon plus 1 teaspoon oil
½ medium onion, diced
1 teaspoon garam masala (see p. 78)
1 teaspoon cumin seeds
½ teaspoon chili powder
2 tablespoons plus 2 teaspoons chopped fresh stalks of coriander
(Chinese parsley)
1 teaspoon salt
2 tomatoes, roughly chopped
fresh coriander leaves, to garnish

Soak dried chickpeas overnight and discard any bad peas.

Cook the chickpeas in a pressure cooker with 1¾ cups water. Continue cooking for 10 minutes after it has pressurized. Drain and reserve the stock for later use. Alternatively, bring chickpeas and water to a boil in an ordinary saucepan and keep at a lively simmer for 1 hour or until soft. If using canned chickpeas, drain and reserve the can liquid.

Heat the oil in a saucepan or wok over low heat, and sauté the onion until it is translucent.

Make a paste of the garam masala, cumin seeds, and chili powder with 1 tablespoon of water. Add the paste to the onions and sauté until fragrant.

Add the coriander stalks, chickpeas, and salt. Stir well, and add the tomatoes. Add 1¼ cups of the reserved chickpea liquid and simmer for 30 to 40 minutes, or until the sauce has reduced by two-thirds. (If using canned chickpeas and there is insufficient liquid, add water or vegetable broth.)

Serve hot, garnished with fresh coriander leaves.

Serves 4 to 6.

*Recipe adapted from an original by Dr. A. Gulati.*

# STIR-FRIED GREEN BEANS WITH PINE NUTS

PER SERVING: 192 CALORIES, 6.8 G PROTEIN, 16.2 G CARBOHYDRATE,
13.9 G FAT (1.6 G SATURATED),490.6 MG SODIUM, 2.6 G FIBER.

1 pound fresh green (string) beans
1 tablespoon plus 1 teaspoon cooking oil (soy, peanut, canola)
2 tablespoons plus 2 teaspoons pine nuts
1 clove garlic, finely diced
1 tablespoon plus 1 teaspoon light soy sauce
1 tablespoon plus 1 teaspoon oyster sauce
½ teaspoon cornstarch
¼ cup water or stock
pinch of ground black pepper (optional)

Rinse the beans and remove ends before cutting each bean into ¾- to 1½-inch lengths. Drain well.

Add 2 drops of oil to a wok over medium heat. Roast the pine nuts for 5 minutes, taking care not to scorch. Remove the pine nuts from the wok and spread out on absorbent kitchen paper to cool.

Heat the remaining oil in the wok over high heat. Sauté the garlic until brown, and then add the beans and stir-fry for a couple of minutes before adding the light soy sauce and oyster sauce. Cover for 1 minute, and uncover to stir well again.

Mix the cornstarch with the water and stir into the wok. Cook for a further 5 minutes.

Stir in the pine nuts and add a dash of pepper (if using) and serve immediately.

Serves 3 to 4.

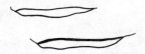

**Note:** This dish goes well with steamed rice, pasta, noodles, or meat.

Fresh beans contain coumestrol and lignans. The concentration of coumestrol in fresh green beans is about the same as that in a similar weight of dried soybeans. However, it is 60 to 70 times less than that present in soybean sprouts. The seedling of the green bean is reported to contain estradiol, a natural estrogen found in women's blood.

# STIR-FRIED PRAWNS, SNOW PEAS, AND TOFU

PER SERVING: 406 CALORIES, 21.6 G PROTEIN, 17.8 G CARBOHYDRATE, 28.1 G FAT (4.1 G SATURATED), 1179.3 MG SODIUM, 2.8 G FIBER.

7 ounces fresh prawns peeled and deveined
2 tablespoons plus 2 teaspoons soy sauce
2 tablespoons plus 2 teaspoons oyster sauce
1 teaspoon Chinese rice wine, dry sherry, or white wine
10 ounces firm tofu
6 tablespoons plus 2 teaspoons cooking oil
4 tablespoons cornstarch
1¼ cups snow peas rinsed and ends trimmed
1 medium onion, peeled and cut into ½-inch strips
¼ cup plus 1 tablespoon chicken stock or canned broth
½ teaspoon salt or to taste
½ teaspoon sugar

Marinate the shrimp in 1 tablespoon plus 1 teaspoon of the soy sauce, 1 tablespoon plus 1 teaspoon of the oyster sauce, and the wine for 10 minutes.

Gently remove the tofu from its package and cut into 1¼- to 1¾-inch cubes. Pat dry with paper towels.

Heat 3 tablespoons plus 1 teaspoon of the cooking oil in a nonstick saucepan and coat the tofu in 2 tablespoons of the cornstarch. When the oil in the pan is smoking, fry the tofu until it is brown on all sides. Remove from the pan, drain off excess oil, and arrange on a serving plate.

In a clean wok or saucepan, heat the remaining oil over medium heat. Stir-fry the marinated shrimp for 3 minutes, and then remove from the wok. Now add the snow peas and onion, and stir-fry together for 4 minutes.

Add the ¼ cup stock, the remaining oyster sauce and soy sauce, and the sugar and salt.

Return the shrimp to the wok. Mix the remaining cornstarch with the 1 tablespoon stock, and add to the shrimp mixture to thicken the sauce. Cook for a further 2 minutes.

Pour the shrimp mixture and its sauce on top of the cooked tofu. Serve with rice or instant noodles.

Serves 4.

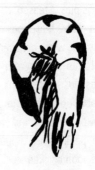

# BEAN SPROUTS IN FISH SAUCE

PER SERVING: 141 CALORIES, 5.4 G PROTEIN, 6.4 G CARBOHYDRATE,
12.3 G FAT (1.8 G SATURATED), 2265.9 MG SODIUM, 1.6 G FIBER.

8 ounces bean sprouts or sprouts, stringy tails trimmed off
1 tablespoon plus 1 teaspoon cooking oil
2 cloves garlic, diced
1 tablespoon plus 1 teaspoon light soy sauce
2 tablespoons plus 2 teaspoons Asian fish sauce (nam pla, nuoc manh, or patis)
1 tablespoon plus 1 teaspoon sesame seeds, lightly toasted
1 small red bell pepper, seeded and shredded, to garnish
fresh coriander (Chinese parsley) leaves, to garnish

Bring 4 cups water to a boil in a medium saucepan.

Blanch the bean sprouts in the boiling water for 30 seconds.
Drain well in a colander.

Discard the water and heat the oil in the saucepan. Add the
garlic and sauté until light brown and fragrant.

Add the light soy sauce and fish sauce. Stir in the blanched
bean sprouts and mix quickly before transferring to a serving dish.

Sprinkle the sesame seeds over the bean sprouts. Garnish with
capsicum and coriander leaves, and serve hot with rice.

Serves 2 to 4.

❖					❖
Fresh bean sprouts cook very quickly and do not tolerate
reheating at all. They are readily available everywhere and also very
cheap. Fresh bean sprouts are sprouted from mung beans and are
quite easy to grow at home. Bean sprouts are very rich in vitamin C,
B-vitamins, and protein, although it is only a second-class protein.
Its phytoestrogens are mainly in the form of lignans and coumestrol. Asian fish sauce (the name varies with the country of origin,
but all are similar) can be found in the Asian foods section of large
supermarkets, as well as in Asian markets, and can be obtained by
mail order.
❖					❖

# CHEESY SCALLOPED POTATOES

PER SERVING: 194 CALORIES, 3.7 G PROTEIN, 27.7 G CARBOHYDRATE,
7.9 G FAT (1.6 G SATURATED), 363.3 MG SODIUM, 2.3 G FIBER.

non-stick vegetable spray
6 medium boiling (thin-skinned) potatoes, unpeeled, scrubbed well and
thinly sliced
½ cup chopped onions
½ cup nonfat milk
1½ cups soy milk
3 tablespoons flour
2 tablespoons soy margarine or butter
1 teaspoon salt or seasoned salt
1 teaspoon parsley flakes
pinch of nutmeg
cayenne to taste
paprika (preferably Hungarian paprika, mild or hot)
1 cup light shredded cheddar cheese

Lightly coat a 9 × 13-inch baking dish with non-stick vegetable spray. Place potato slices and onions in dish.

In a saucepan, combine the nonfat milk, soy milk, flour, margarine, salt, parsley flakes, nutmeg, and paprika or cayenne. Heat,
stirring constantly, until slightly thickened. Stir in cheese and
pour over potatoes, mixing well. Lightly dust paprika over the top.

Cover with foil and cook at 350°F for 1 hour. Remove cover
and cook another 15 minutes until brown.

Serves 8.

*Recipe from* It's Soy Easy…to Cook with Soy. *By permission of the
Ohio Soybean Council.*

# FRIED RICE

PER SERVING: 397 CALORIES, 15.6 G PROTEIN, 53.5 G CARBOHYDRATE,
12.7 G FAT (1.2 G SATURATED), 1063.5 MG SODIUM, 2.9 G FIBER.

1 large egg
pinch of salt
freshly ground black pepper, to taste
2 tablespoons plus 2 teaspoons cooking oil (soybean, peanut, or canola)
1 tablespoon plus 1 teaspoon diced onion
4 ounces Chinese barbecued pork (char siew) or packaged lean honey ham, cut into
¼-inch cubes (see note below)
1 cup frozen green peas, rinsed and drained
3 cups cooked long-grain rice, fully cooled
4 tablespoons light soy sauce
1 tablespoon plus 1 teaspoon oyster sauce
3 cooked shrimp or prawns, peeled, deveined, and diced (optional)
1 medium carrot, shredded
fresh coriander (Chinese parsley, cilantro) leaves, to garnish (optional)

Beat the egg with the salt and pepper to taste.

Heat ½ tablespoon of the oil in a wok over medium heat. When the oil is hot, add the beaten egg and spread the egg over the bottom of the wok as if cooking a thin crêpe. As soon as the egg is cooked, remove from the pan—do not overcook the egg, as this will make it rubbery. Allow to cool before cutting into ½- to 1-inch strips. Set aside.

Heat the remaining soybean oil in the wok. Add the onion and sauté until fragrant and just starting to brown.

Add the pork (see note) and green peas, and stir-fry for 1 minute. Add the rice and mix well, stirring constantly. Add the soy sauce and oyster sauce, and mix well.

Cook for another 5 minutes, and then make a hollow in the middle of the rice. Add the carrot and the shrimp (if using) to the hollow. Continue stir-frying for another 5 minutes.

Add the shredded egg and mix well through the fried rice. Garnish with the coriander leaves (if using) and serve hot.

Serves 4 to 6.

**Note:** This recipe is easily adapted for low-fat and vegetarian diets. Instead of the barbecued pork you can substitute 1¾ ounces of diced light ham; vegetarians can use 3½ ounces of tofu cutlet, diced into small cubes, or smoked soy "meat."

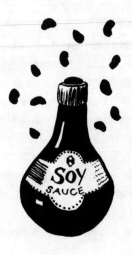

# Main Courses

Gado Gado

Hot Pot (Steamboat)

Poached Spiced Chicken

Spiced Roast Chicken

Teriyaki Chicken

Sesame Chicken Fillet

Chicken Breasts with
  Chipotle Sauce

Tacos

Festive Vegetable Fajita Wraps

Healthy Chilii

Curried Tofu and Vegetables

Vegetable Tofu Stir-Fry

Tofu in Oyster Sauce

Hunanese Tofu Beef

Tofu with Ground Meat

Steamed Fish with Tofu

Sweet and Sour Tofu

Corn Bread Tamale Pie

Stewed Bean Curd Skin and
  Cloud Ears with Pork

Stir-Fried Tempeh and Vegetables

Tofu Cutlet in Lettuce Leaves
  with Prawns

Soybean Sprouts with Ground Pork

Soybean Sprouts with Shredded
  Beef

Soybean Sprouts with Shrimp

Baked Soybeans in Eggplant

Stir-Fried Rice Noodles

Stir-Fried Chinese Cabbage
  and Bean Thread Noodles

Mediterranean Spinach Pasta

Sesame Tofu and Spinach Pasta

Easy Vegetable Lasagna

Tuna Soy-Mac Casserole

# GADO GADO

PER SERVING: 317 CALORIES, 15.4 G PROTEIN, 20.7 G CARBOHYDRATE,
18.1 G FAT (2.2 G SATURATED), 789.1 MG SODIUM, 5.9 G FIBER.

1 tablespoon plus 1 teaspoon cooking oil (soybean, peanut, or canola)
10 ounces firm tofu, cut into cubes
3½ ounces tempeh, sliced
6 ounces green beans (string beans), trimmed
2 tablespoons plus 2 teaspoons hot water
4 tablespoons ketjap manis (see Glossary)
2 teaspoons garlic, finely diced
2 tablespoons plus 2 teaspoons Asian chili sauce (see Glossary)
5 tablespoons plus 1 teaspoon crushed roasted peanuts
1½ cup jicama
1 11-ounce can pineapple pieces
2 medium tomatoes
2 cucumbers
8 ounces mung bean sprouts, stringy tail portions removed
(Heads may be snapped off if desired; the sprouts will taste better
but have lower nutritional value.)

Heat the oil in non-stick frying pan or skillet. Fry the tofu and
tempeh until the skin is brown and crispy. Drain on paper towels.

Drop green beans into boiling salted water to cover. Blanch
until crisp-tender (2-3 minutes, depending on thickness). Immediately
drain and run under cold water until cool. Drain again.

Mix the hot water, ketjap manis, garlic, chili sauce, and peanuts
in a soup or small serving bowl. This is the gado gado sauce.

Using a sturdy paring knife, peel the jicama (if using) and cut
into strips like potato chips or thick-cut French fries. Cut the
pineapple, tomatoes, and cucumbers into bite-size chunks.

Boil some water and blanch the bean sprouts for a minute.
Drain well and arrange the green beans, jicama, pineapple, tomatoes,
cucumber, and bean sprouts on a platter with the tofu and
tempeh.

Serve cold accompanied by the gado gado sauce. Each person selects from the platter and then pours some gado gado sauce over the top of their food.

Serves 6 to 8.

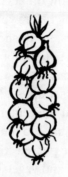

❖ This dish goes well with coconut-flavored rice and fish, or plain rice with curries. Green beans contain phytoestrogens.

# HOT POT (STEAMBOAT)

Steamboat, the Australian name for Mongolian Hot Pot, is particularly good in cold weather and whenever you want to linger over a meal, chatting with your fellow diners between the various courses and watching the dishes cook before your very eyes at the dining table. Diners cook vegetables, meat, and seafood in broth at the table, adding various sauces to their food, and then they drink the soup remaining in the cooker.

A hot pot is not hard to set up. A Mongolian cooker on charcoal is traditionally placed at the center of the table, with insulation adequate to prevent damage to the table. If you do not have a Mongolian hot pot, a fondue pot, electric rice cooker, or electric wok will do just fine. Meats and vegetables are cooked in stock, and special wire-mesh nets are used to fish the items out. These nets are cheap and easily obtained from most Asian grocery stores and from cookwares stores and catalogs such as Williams Sonoma and Sur La Table.

Seafood cooks quite quickly in rapidly boiling stock, while meats such as pork and chicken take longer. Pork takes the longest time to cook. Slicing meats thinly will ensure shorter cooking times. All the vegetables and the tofu listed in this recipe cook very quickly. The bean thread noodles will take about twice as long as the vegetables to cook.

The various sauces (recipes follow) are placed around the table in places that diners can easily reach; some sauces go better with certain meats or vegetables. Here are some suggestions of what goes with what:

**Fragrant soy sauce:** Practically all the meats and vegetables listed in this recipe go very well with this sauce.

**Oyster sauce:** Meats and scallops go well with oyster sauce. Chinese cabbage, tofu, Chinese chrysanthemums, and bean sprouts also taste great with it.

**Satay peanut sauce:** All meats and vegetables go with this sauce. However, some items, such as squid, beef, chicken, bean sprouts, tofu, and shrimp, taste exceptionally delicious with this sauce.

**Lime and fish sauce:** Seafood such as shrimp (prawns), fish, and scallops are suggested for this sauce. Chicken is also suitable.

**Plum sauce:** All meats go well with this sauce. Perhaps surprisingly, fish tastes good with plum sauce, too.

**Hoisin sauce:** This sauce goes very well with tofu and beef. Try it with squid and pork as well.

**Tom yum sauce:** This hot and tangy sauce goes well with any of the meats and vegetables listed in this recipe, if you do not mind the sauce's heat. It's normally used with seafood.

**Asian Chili sauce:** This sauce goes well with any meat or seafood. Bean sprouts can be eaten with chili sauce if you like your food hot.

You will notice that we've given no calculation of the nutritional content of this recipe. Because this is a versatile dish (you can use any combination of vegetables, meats, sauces, and seafoods), it is impossible to calculate values for the mixture of ingredients that you will use. In practical terms, the meats and vegetables and other items used in this recipe don't fit standard serving sizes anyway. You simply select what you like in the amount that you like, with whatever sauces you like.

1 pound fresh shrimp or prawns, peeled and deveined

10 ounces scallops

7 ounces lean boneless pork, very thinly sliced

7 ounces boneless beef, very thinly sliced

10 ounces skinned, boned chicken breast, very thinly sliced

10 ounces cleaned squid, cut into bite-size pieces

10 ounces meatballs, halved

fresh coriander (Chinese parsley) leaves or similar herbs, to garnish

3½ ounces bean thread noodles

¾ cup Chinese (Nappa) cabbage

1 bunch of Chinese chrysanthemum vegetable

1 bunch of green onions

8 ounces bean sprouts

1¼ pounds tofu

3 to 4 quarts chicken stock (p. 77) or canned chicken broth

Wash and salt the shrimp very lightly. Wash the scallops, drain them, and set aside with just a pinch of salt.

Arrange all the meat and seafood on a platter and garnish with coriander or similar herbs. Store in the refrigerator until ready to use.

Soak the bean thread noodles in cold water. Drain well before use. Rinse the Chinese cabbage and cut into bite-size pieces. Drain well.

Rinse and drain the Chinese chrysanthemum vegetable very well, as there is usually a lot of soil caught between its leaves.

Cut the spring onions into 1¼- to 1¾-inch lengths and wash well. Rinse the bean sprouts and trim the roots if necessary.

Arrange the vegetables and tofu on another platter with the bean vermicelli. Place on the table with the meat and seafood platter.

Pour 2 to 3 liters of the stock into the cooker and bring to a boil. Cook the items one group at a time to ensure complete and even cooking. For example, beef cooks faster than pork, and bean sprouts cook faster than Chinese cabbage. Use wire-mesh nets to remove the cooked items from the stock.

Eat while hot, dipping individual items into any of the sauces listed below. Top the "steamboat" up with more stock if necessary. Serves 6 to 8.

### Fragrant Soy Sauce

Sauté 1 tablespoon plus 1 teaspoon diced onion and 1 tablespoon plus 1 teaspoon diced garlic in 1 tablespoon plus 1 teaspoon soybean oil until golden brown. Add a pinch of sugar, 2 tablespoons plus 2 teaspoons hot water, and ⅓ cup light soy sauce.

### Oyster Sauce

Add 2 teaspoons sesame oil to 2 tablespoons plus 2 teaspoons good-quality oyster sauce, and then mix with 3 teaspoons hot water.

### Lime and Fish Sauce

Shred 3 to 4 young lime leaves and 1 red chili pepper. Combine with 2 tablespoons plus 2 teaspoons fish sauce, 1 tablespoon plus

2 teaspoons lime juice, 1 teaspoon sugar, and 2 tablespoons plus 2 teaspoons hot water.

### Plum Sauce

Mix 1 tablespoon plus 1 teaspoon plum sauce with 1 tablespoon plus 1 teaspoon hot water and ¼ teaspoon salt.

### Hoisin Sauce

Mix 1 tablespoon plus 1 teaspoon hoi sin sauce with 5 teaspoons hot water and 1 teaspoon sesame oil.

### Tom Yum Sauce

Mix 1 tablespoon plus 1 teaspoon tom yum paste with 2 tablespoons plus 2 teaspoons hot water, 2 teaspoons lime juice, ¼ teaspoon salt, and 1 teaspoon sugar.

### Chili Sauce

Blend ½ cup hot chili peppers, 2 cloves garlic, 1 teaspoon chopped fresh ginger, 1 teaspoon sugar, and ¾ teaspoon salt in 2 to 2½ tablespoons white vinegar. Alternatively, use one of the commercial brands of ready-made Asian chili sauce.

### Satay Peanut Sauce

Sauté 1 tablespoon plus 1 teaspoon diced garlic and 1 tablespoon plus 1 teaspoon diced onion in 1 tablespoon plus 1 teaspoon oil. Add 2 teaspoons curry powder mixed with 2 tablespoons chicken stock or canned broth. Add 2 finely crushed macadamia nuts and, if available, 6 curry leaves. Sauté until fragrant, and then add 1¼ cups canned unsweetened coconut milk (well-stirred), ½ teaspoon lime juice, and ½ teaspoon sugar.

Bring to a boil, and then remove from the heat and add ½ cup shelled, peeled, and crushed roasted peanuts.

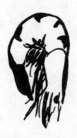

# POACHED SPICED CHICKEN

PER SERVING: 345 CALORIES, 69.1 G PROTEIN, 15.9 G CARBOHYDRATE,
16.2 G FAT (0 G SATURATED), 5536.9 MG SODIUM, .1 G FIBER.

4 cups water

scant 1 cup light soy sauce

scant 1 cup dark soy sauce

1 tablespoon plus 1 teaspoon sugar

2 cloves garlic

2 pieces licorice root (see note)

1 stick cinnamon

1 star anise (see note)

10 black peppercorns

1 tablespoon plus 1 teaspoon oyster sauce

1 tablespoon plus 1 teaspoon Chinese rice wine (Shao Hsing Chiew), dry sherry,
or white wine

¾-inch piece fresh ginger

4 leg-thigh pieces chicken

Optional garnishes: sliced cucumber, sliced tomatoes, fresh coriander leaf (cilantro)

Bring all the ingredients except the chicken to a boil in a
medium-size saucepan. Allow to boil for 5 minutes.

Trim any visible fat off the chicken and discard. (Chicken may
be skinned if desired to decrease fat.) Pat the chicken dry with
absorbent kitchen paper or a clean cloth.

Gently lower the chicken into the boiling stock. Bring the liquid to a boil once again, and then turn off the heat, cover with lid,
and let stand for 15 minutes on the stove. Turn the chicken pieces
over in the saucepan and once again bring just to boiling. Cover and
turn off the heat once more and let stand for another 15 minutes.

Test whether the chicken is cooked by inserting a fork into the
meaty part of the thigh. If it is cooked, the juices will run clear
with no tinge of pink.

Serve hot with potatoes or steamed rice. Garnish with sliced
cucumber, tomatoes, and fresh coriander, if desired.

Serves 4.

**Note:** If you can't find star anise and licorice root, use a teaspoon of Chinese five-spice powder, found in the spice section of large supermarkets, and easily available from mail order spice catalogs.

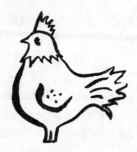

The stock can be made ahead of time and frozen until you are ready to use it. Simply thaw it and continue with the recipe as above. Beef can be used instead of chicken. You can also use other parts or cuts of chicken, such as wings, thighs, or breast filets, but the nutritional information will differ from those given above.

❖ Licorice has very potent antiflushing effects. It can be used ❖
in infusion as a beverage. The root is quite sweet and is sold sliced
in plastic bags. It may be found in Asian markets and herbal phar-
macies, and is available by mail order. People suffering from high
blood pressure should not use licorice.
❖                                                                   ❖

# SPICED ROAST CHICKEN

PER SERVING: 280 CALORIES, 64.5 G PROTEIN, 5 G CARBOHYDRATE, 16.2 G FAT (0 G SATURATED), 792.3 MG SODIUM, .4 G FIBER.

2 leg-thigh pieces of chicken
2 tablespoons plus 2 teaspoons light soy sauce
½ teaspoon dried sage
1 teaspoon ground fennel
½ teaspoon ground cinnamon
¼ teaspoon star anise powder
¼ teaspoon ground black pepper
½ teaspoon sugar
2 cloves garlic, finely chopped

Remove any visible fat from the chicken. Pat the chicken dry with paper towels.

Place the chicken in a container suitable for marinating and add the remaining ingredients. Marinate in the refrigerator for at least 4 hours, preferably overnight, turning the chicken pieces occasionally to coat all sides evenly.

Preheat the oven to 325°F. Place the marinated chicken on a rack in a roasting pan and roast for 40 minutes. Baste the skin with the remaining marinade at least once during the roasting time. Chicken may also be broiled or barbecued. Check doneness by puncturing the thigh; if juices run clear with no pink tinge, chicken is ready.

Serve hot with vegetables and noodles.

Serves 2.

❖                                                                    ❖
Sage, fennel, and cinnamon all contain phytoestrogens.
Soy sauce is made from fermented soybeans and contains very small quantities of phytoestrogens. The oil and fat in this dish drain off during cooking if the chicken is roasted on a rack. If you wish to reduce the fat content of this dish even further, remove the chicken's skin before marinating.

❖                                                                    ❖

# TERIYAKI CHICKEN

PER SERVING: 650 CALORIES, 130.2 G PROTEIN, 11.9 G CARBOHYDRATE,
41 G FAT (1.3 G SATURATED), 2905 MG SODIUM, .1 G FIBER.

14 ounces chicken thigh, skinned and boned (or chicken breast or fish fillet)
¼ teaspoon sugar
pinch of salt
5 tablespoons plus 1 teaspoon teriyaki sauce
1 tablespoon plus 1 teaspoon sesame oil, for basting
lettuce leaves, to garnish

Remove any visible fat from the chicken and discard. Slice the meat into strips ¾-inch thick and place in a bowl.

Sprinkle the sugar and salt over the chicken and mix well. Add the teriyaki sauce and let marinate in the refrigerator for at least 30 minutes.

Cook on a hot grill or under the broiler, turning the chicken after 5 minutes. Baste with any remaining marinade and the sesame oil.

Serve hot on a bed of lettuce leaves.

Serves 2 to 4.

**Note:** This dish goes very well with rice and stir-fried or steamed vegetables. Other accompaniments, such as raw vegetable salads or pickled radish, ginger, and carrots, can be served with the rice.

❖ Skinned, boned chicken breast can be used instead of thigh; it has much less fat. Fish filets can be used in place of chicken. In either case, these take less cooking time than chicken thigh, so check each side after two minutes and take care not to overcook. When the meat feels springy to the touch, it is done. Teriyaki sauce is made from soybeans and also contains wine, wheat, and spices. ❖

# SESAME CHICKEN FILLET

PER SERVING: 828 CALORIES, 161.9 G PROTEIN, 9.3 G CARBOHYDRATE,
55.2 G FAT (2.2 G SATURATED), 951.7 MG SODIUM, 2.6 G FIBER.

1 pound skinned and boned chicken thighs (or 1½ pounds bone-in)
1 tablespoon plus 1 teaspoon Chinese rice wine or dry sherry
1 tablespoon plus 1 teaspoon light soy sauce
1 tablespoon plus 1 teaspoon oyster sauce
1 clove garlic, diced
1 tablespoon plus 1 teaspoon tahini (see Glossary)
1¼-inch piece of fresh ginger, peeled, thinly sliced
2 teaspoons sesame oil
2 tablespoons plus 2 teaspoons sesame seeds
¼ teaspoon salt

Trim and discard any visible fat from the chicken. Cut the
chicken into bite-size chunks. Place chicken, wine, soy sauce, oyster sauce, garlic, and tahini in a bowl, and marinate in the refrigerator for 1 hour.

Heat the sesame oil in a wok over medium heat and stir-fry the
sliced ginger until fragrant.

Increase the heat, add the marinated chicken and stir-fry until
no moist sauce is left in the wok (10-15 minutes).

Reduce the heat (to medium) and add the sesame seeds. (The
sesame seeds need to be stir-fried over moderate heat or they may
burn or jump out of the wok.)

Serve with steamed vegetables and rice.

Serves 2 to 4.

❖ This dish is traditionally cooked for new mothers using much
more ginger. The dish's nutritional and estrogen content helps to
buffer a woman from the rapid plunge in natural estrogen levels
that follows the birth of a baby. Phytoestrogens are present in
whole sesame seeds, sesame oil, and tahini. Fresh ginger contains a
natural anticoagulant that helps prevent deep venous thrombosis
and pulmonary embolism (clots in the legs and lungs). ❖

# CHICKEN BREASTS
# WITH CHIPOTLE SAUCE

PER SERVING: 248 CALORIES, 20.4 G PROTEIN, 15 G CARBOHYDRATE, 9 G FAT (1.6 G SATURATED), 255.6 MG SODIUM, 3.4 G FIBER.

2 whole chicken breasts, skinned and halved

1 small onion

1 small carrot

1 small celery stalk with leaves

6 whole black peppercorns

3 cups chicken stock (p. 77) or canned low-salt chicken broth

3 tomatoes, peeled and diced for garnish

2 green onion stems (green part only), finely chopped

### Sauce:
additional ¾ cup chicken stock

¾ cup mashed silken tofu

generous ¼ cup minced onion

3 tablespoons canned chipotle chiles in adobo sauce, sauce scraped off, seeded

3 tablespoons peanut butter (any type on hand)

salt to taste

Combine chicken, onion, carrot, celery, and peppercorns in a large heavy saucepan. Add enough stock to cover chicken. Bring to a boil. Skim gray foam from the surface and immediately remove pan from the heat, cover, and let stand until the chicken is springy to the touch, about 15 minutes.

While chicken is poaching, make sauce: Puree all sauce ingredients in a food processor or blender until smooth. Pour into a heavy medium saucepan and bring to a simmer. Stir over low heat for five minutes. Pour through a strainer into another pan or a pyrex measuring cup, pressing on the sieve with the back of a spoon. If too thick, stir in additional stock (from the poaching liquid). Adjust seasoning and cover to keep warm.

Drain chicken breasts well, reserving stock for another use. Place chicken breasts on serving plates and spoon sauce over them. (For a dressier presentation, lift meat carefully off the bone, slice, and arrange in a fan on each plate.) Sprinkle with tomatoes and green onions and serve immediately.

This very spicy dish calls for rice and warmed tortillas to accompany it, along with a vegetable or salad.

Serves 4.

*Recipe from Naomi Wise.*

# TACOS

PER SERVING: 355 CALORIES, 14.6 G PROTEIN, 35.2 G CARBOHYDRATE,
18.4 G FAT (4.3 G SATURATED), 511.1 MG SODIUM, 6.9 G FIBER.

1 pound tofu, crumbled
2 tablespoons cooking oil (soy, peanut, canola)
1 package taco seasoning
½ cup water
6 corn tortillas, warmed
1 can refried beans of choice, heated
tomatoes, chopped
lettuce, chopped
green onions, chopped
salsa of choice

In a large saucepan, cook tofu over medium heat for about 10 minutes. Add the taco seasoning and water to the saucepan. Cook until the sauce is thick and the tofu is completely cooked.

To serve, spread each tortilla with a generous layer of refried beans. Add several heaping spoonfuls of tofu. Sprinkle with chopped tomato, lettuce, and scallions. Top with salsa.

Serves 6.

*Recipe courtesy of the Indiana Soybean Board.*

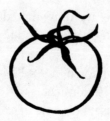

# FESTIVE VEGETABLE
# FAJITA WRAPS

PER SERVING: 129 CALORIES, 10.3 G PROTEIN, 13.4 G CARBOHYDRATE,
4.6 G FAT (1.1 G SATURATED), 97.8 MG SODIUM, 2.5 G FIBER.

### Filling:

1½ cups cooked soybeans (see p. 76)
½ cup chopped red onion
½ cup chopped green bell pepper
½ cup chopped yellow, red, or orange pepper
1 chile such as jalapeño or serrano (seeds and ribs removed)
1 chipotle chile (very hot)
2 tablespoons lime juice
2 tablespoons chopped fresh cilantro
½ teaspoon chopped fresh garlic
¼ teaspoon cumin
½ cup lowfat shredded cheddar cheese

### Shells:

8 soft corn or flour tortilla shells
bean sprouts (garnish to taste)

### Garnishes:

salsa, guacamole, low-fat sour cream

In a large bowl, combine filling ingredients and mix well.
Spoon filling across center of shells and top with bean sprouts.
Roll up.

To warm, place seam down in 9 × 12-inch baking dish, bake
uncovered at 350°F for 10 minutes.

Serve fajitas with salsa, guacamole, or low-fat sour cream.
Serves 8.

Note: For a different twist, add 1 cup sliced grilled chicken or beef
and 4 ounces of Monterey Jack cheese to the filling.

*Recipe from* It's Soy Easy…to Cook with Soy. *By permission of the*
*Ohio Soybean Council.*

# HEALTHY CHILI

PER SERVING: 582 CALORIES, 24.9 G PROTEIN, 92 G CARBOHYDRATE,
15.4 G FAT (2.2 G SATURATED), 1139.3 MG SODIUM, 14.2 G FIBER.

2 cups firm tofu, crumbled

1 clove garlic, minced

1 tablespoon chili powder

2 tablespoons Worchestershire sauce

1 cup onion, chopped

1 large green pepper, chopped

1 carrot, thinly sliced

2 tablespoons cooking oil

1 cup tomatoes, chopped

1 16-ounce can tomato sauce

1 15-ounce can dark red kidney beans

1 teaspoon dried basil, crushed

1 teaspoon cumin

1 teaspoon cayenne pepper

1 6-ounce can tomato paste, optional

salt to taste

4 cups cooked brown or white rice

**Garnishes:**

minced onion, grated cheddar cheese, avocado (optional)

In a mixing bowl, combine tofu, garlic, chili powder, and Worchestershire sauce; set aside.

In a large skillet, sauté onion, green pepper, and carrot in oil until onion becomes transparent. Add tofu mixture, stir in and cook for 3 minutes over medium heat. Add tomatoes, tomato sauce, kidney beans, basil, cumin, cayenne, and, if desired, tomato paste. Cover and simmer for 30 minutes. Salt to taste. (If there is time, refrigerate overnight to blend flavors, then reheat gently.) Serve over brown or white rice. Garnish if desired.

Serves 8.

*Recipe used courtesy of the Indiana Soybean Board.*

# CURRIED TOFU AND VEGETABLES

PER SERVING: 556 CALORIES, 31.1 G PROTEIN, 32.4 G CARBOHYDRATE,
35.3 G FAT (10.8 G SATURATED), 424.7 MG SODIUM, 8.1 G FIBER.

1 tablespoon plus 1 teaspoon cooking oil (soy, canola, olive)
4 tablespoons diced onion or ½ large onion, diced
¾-inch piece of fresh ginger, diced
1 tablespoon plus 1 teaspoon curry powder
1¼ cup chicken stock (p. 77), canned chicken broth, or vegetable broth
10 ounces pumpkin or any winter squash, peeled and cut into ¾- to 1-inch cubes
1½ cups green (string) beans, trimmed and cut into 1- to 1¼-inch lengths
7 ounces fried or baked tofu (see p. 79)
1 eggplant, preferably long, narrow Asian eggplant, about 7 to 10 ounces,
cut into ¾- to 1-inch cubes
2 macadamia nuts, ground (or substitute 6 cashews or almonds)
5 tablespoons plus 1 teaspoon shredded unsweetened coconut
½ teaspoon salt or to taste

Heat the oil in a medium saucepan over medium heat. Sauté
the onion and ginger for 2 minutes.

Meanwhile, mix the curry powder and ¼ cup water into a
paste. Add to the onion mixture and sauté for another 2 to 3 minutes, or until very fragrant.

Add the pumpkin or squash and stir for a few minutes. Then
add the green beans, tofu, and eggplant. Add 1 cup broth and the
nuts, coconut, and salt to taste. Simmer for 20 to 25 minutes.
Serve hot with rice, bread, or noodles.

Serves 4 to 6.

Note: Fresh shelled and deveined shrimp (prawns) can be added 8
to 10 minutes before the end of the cooking time if desired.

❖ The best result is obtained with ready-fried tofu (see pp. 73
and 79). If you are worried about the fat content, use hard tofu.
Grill it on both sides (see p. 80) until light brown before using
in the above recipe. ❖

# VEGETABLE TOFU STIR-FRY

PER SERVING: 148 CALORIES, 10.2 G PROTEIN, 11.1 G CARBOHYDRATE,
8.5 G FAT (1.2 G SATURATED), 715.4 MG SODIUM, 3.8 G FIBER.

1 tablespoon vegetable oil
1 teaspoon peeled minced ginger
1 clove garlic, minced
14 ounces extra-firm tofu,* drained and cut into ¾-inch cubes
1 cup broccoli florets
1 small red bell pepper, diced
1 large carrot, grated
¼ cup water chestnuts
1 tablespoon light soy sauce
1 tablespoon oyster sauce
1 teaspoon salt
⅛ teaspoon pepper

*Azumaya or other brand

Heat oil in a non-stick skillet over medium heat. Add ginger
and garlic and sauté 1 minute. Add tofu and sauté until lightly
browned, 3 to 5 minutes.

Add remaining vegetables and sauté 2 minutes. Add soy sauce,
oyster sauce, salt, and pepper; sauté and gently stir to heat. Serve
over a bed of rice.

Serves 4.

*Recipe from* Delicious and Easy Recipes for Tofu and Pasta. *By permission
of Azumaya.*

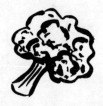

# TOFU IN OYSTER SAUCE

PER SERVING: 195 CALORIES, 6.3 G PROTEIN, 11.2 G CARBOHYDRATE,
14.3 G FAT (0 G SATURATED), 738.2 MG SODIUM, .5 G FIBER.

10 ounces silken tofu

2 tablespoons plus 2 teaspoons soybean oil

1 clove garlic, diced

1 small red onion, diced

2 tablespoons plus 2 teaspoons oyster sauce (see Glossary)

1 tablespoon plus 1 teaspoon light soy sauce

¼ cup chicken stock (p. 77) or broth, or vegetable broth

freshly ground black pepper, to taste

½ teaspoon cornstarch

fresh coriander (Chinese parsley) or celery leaves, to garnish

Cut the tofu into 6 pieces.

Heat the soybean oil in a wok and stir-fry the garlic and onion until fragrant. Remove from the wok and set aside.

Now stir-fry the tofu; be gentle, as it breaks up very easily. When golden brown in color, transfer the tofu to a serving dish.

Reduce the heat to very low. Return the garlic and onion to the wok, and add the oyster sauce, light soy sauce, chicken stock, pepper to taste, and cornstarch, stirring constantly.

Bring to a boil and immediately pour the sauce over the cooked tofu. Garnish with fresh coriander or celery leaves.

Serve hot, accompanied by steamed rice and stir-fried vegetable dishes.

Serves 3 to 4.

# HUNANESE TOFU BEEF

PER SERVING: 1947 CALORIES, 41 G PROTEIN, 15.3 G CARBOHYDRATE,
192.5 G FAT (35.3 G SATURATED), 995.4 MG SODIUM, 4.2 G FIBER.

1 pound firm fresh tofu

generous ½ cup finely diced carrots or green beans

4 large garlic cloves, smashed with the side of a cleaver and peeled

1 large green onion

1 walnut-size lump fresh ginger, peeled

½ cup rich chicken stock (p. 77) or low-salt canned broth

2 tablespoons light soy sauce

1 tablespoon Chinese rice wine (Shao Hsing) or dry sherry

3–4 cups soy, peanut, or canola oil for frying

6 ounces lean ground beef (from the round)

1 tablespoon Asian chili sauce

¼ teaspoon sugar

¼ teaspoon salt (or to taste)

1½ teaspoons cornstarch dissolved in 1½ tablespoons chicken stock or water

black pepper to taste

Cut tofu into small cubes (about ½-inch square) and spread on paper towels to dry for a few minutes. Meanwhile, blanch the diced carrots or beans in boiling water to cover (about 20 seconds). Drain immediately and refresh under cold water. Let drain. Mince garlic, green onion, and ginger (this may be done in a food processor) and set aside, or refrigerate if you will be completing the dish several hours later. Mix chicken stock, soy sauce, and rice wine, and set aside.

Heat a wok or large heavy skillet until hot. Add oil and heat it to 400°F. Being careful of spattering oil, drop the cubes one by one into the oil and fry until golden (1-2 minutes), gently nudging the cubes apart with a spoon if they stick together. With a mesh strainer or slotted spoon, scoop tofu cubes from the oil and drain well on paper towels, blotting on all sides. (This may be done several hours in advance.) When the oil cools, strain it into a bottle and refrigerate it for future use. (It may be re-used for stir-frying.)

Heat a wok or large skillet, add 3 tablespoons oil, and coat the pan. Add the garlic mixture, lower the heat a little, and stir-fry about 30 seconds (do not allow to brown). Add the meat, breaking it apart and breaking up clumps with chopsticks or the front edge of a metal spatula. Stir-fry over medium-high heat until meat changes color, then stir in chili sauce and vegetables. Pour the soy sauce mixture into the pan. Gently stir in the tofu cubes and bring the mixture to a simmer. Add sugar, salt, and pepper to taste. Lower the heat to medium. Stir the cornstarch mixture again and then stir it into the wok until the sauce thickens slightly. Serve over rice.

Serves 2 as a main dish.

*Recipe from Naomi Wise.*

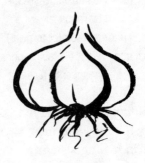

# TOFU WITH GROUND MEAT

PER SERVING: 316 CALORIES, 20.7 G PROTEIN, 21.0 G CARBOHYDRATE,
16.1 G FAT (4.2 G SATURATED), 1088.4 MG SODIUM, .1 G FIBER.

3½ ounces lean ground meat (pork, beef, lamb, or turkey)
1 tablespoon plus 1 teaspoon light soy sauce
1 tablespoon plus 1 teaspoon oyster sauce
1 teaspoon Chinese rice wine or dry sherry
2 tablespoons plus 2 teaspoons cornstarch
freshly ground black pepper, to taste
1 teaspoon cooking oil
1 clove garlic, finely diced
10 ounces silken tofu, cut into ½-inch cubes
1 tablespoon plus 1 teaspoon dark soy sauce
¼ cup water
¼ teaspoon sugar or to taste
pinch of salt (optional)
fresh coriander (Chinese parsley) leaves or spring onion stems, to garnish

Marinate the meat with the light soy sauce, oyster sauce, wine, 1 tablespoon plus 1 teaspoon of the cornstarch, and pepper to taste.

Heat the soybean oil in a wok or frying pan until nearly smoking. Add the garlic and sauté until fragrant, and then add the meat and its marinade. Cook the meat for 4 to 5 minutes over high heat.

Add the tofu and dark soy sauce. Cover the wok and allow to cook for 2 to 3 minutes.

Mix the remaining cornstarch and the water into a paste and add to the wok. Bring to a boil to allow the sauce to thicken.

Taste for the seasoning and add sugar and salt as needed.

Garnish with fresh coriander or spring onion stems, and serve hot with boiled rice.

Serves 2 to 4.

❖ ❖

This is a popular Cantonese dish that is easy to prepare and cook. Ground pork is normally used, but julienne-cut beef or chicken breast fillets can be substituted, resulting in different flavors. An accompanying dish such as steamed vegetables or a stir-fried combination is most suitable.

❖ ❖

# STEAMED FISH WITH TOFU

PER SERVING: 204 CALORIES, 19.7 G PROTEIN, 10.5 G CARBOHYDRATE,
9.3 G FAT (.5 G SATURATED), 567.3 MG SODIUM, .2 G FIBER.

7 ounces firm boneless white fish fillet, such as ling cod, rock cod, sea bass
1 tablespoon plus 1 teaspoon oyster sauce
1 tablespoon plus 1 teaspoon soy sauce
1 teaspoon Chinese rice wine (Shao Hsing) or dry sherry
12 slices fresh ginger
1 tablespoon plus 1 teaspoon cornstarch
3 teaspoons cooking oil (soy, peanut, canola)
1 clove garlic, diced
10 ounces silken firm tofu
green onion or coriander (Chinese parsley) leaves, to garnish

Cut the fish fillet lengthwise into pieces ½-inch thick. Run your fingers carefully over all surfaces of the fish, and use needle-nosed pliers to yank out any bones you find.

Place in a suitable dish with the oyster sauce, soy sauce, wine, ginger, and cornstarch. Marinate in the refrigerator for 20 to 30 minutes.

Heat the oil in a saucepan and sauté the garlic until light brown. Set aside to cool.

Cut the tofu into sheets ½-inch thick. Brush a heatproof ceramic dish lightly with the cooled garlic oil, and layer the tofu over the bottom of the dish.

Place portions of the fish filet on top of each tofu piece. Brush the top of the fish with more of the garlic oil and place a ginger slice on top of each portion.

Pour about ½ inch of water into the bottom of a steamer or a deep large saucepan or covered roaster that will accommodate a rack. Place the dish in the steamer or on the rack. Cover, bring the water rapidly to a boil, and steam the fish for 10 minutes.

Garnish with spring onion or coriander leaves, and serve hot with steamed rice.

Serves 3 to 4.

Whole fish, such as, snapper, rock cod, or black cod can be steamed with tofu, but score the sides of the fish before marinating. Make sure your tofu is fresh; otherwise the dish will turn sourish in taste.

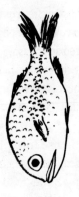

# SWEET AND SOUR TOFU

PER SERVING: 382 CALORIES, 10.4 G PROTEIN, 40.1 G CARBOHYDRATE,
22.5 G FAT (2.8 G SATURATED), 716.3 MG SODIUM, 3.1 G FIBER.

10 ounces silken firm tofu
2 tablespoons plus 2 teaspoons cooking oil, divided
½ medium carrot, julienned
2 tablespoons plus 2 teaspoons apple cider vinegar
1 medium onion, sliced
½ teaspoon salt
2 tablespoons plus 2 teaspoons tomato sauce or ketchup
¾ cup cucumber, cut into chunks
½ cup pineapple pieces, cut into chunks
½ medium red bell pepper, cut into chunks
1 tablespoon plus 1 teaspoon sugar
freshly ground black pepper, to taste
½ teaspoon cornstarch
2 tablespoons water

Cut the tofu into ¾-inch cubes. Heat 1 tablespoon plus 1 teaspoon of the oil in a wok and fry the tofu cubes until they are golden brown on all sides, turning gently to brown all sides.

Marinate the carrot in the cider vinegar. Cut the onions into strips by sectioning each into 8 wedges and separating into pieces. Sauté the onion in the remaining soybean oil for 2 minutes, and then add the carrot and the apple cider vinegar in which it was marinated.

Add the salt, tomato sauce, cucumber, pineapple, and bell pepper. Stir well, then add the sugar and pepper to taste. Mix the cornstarch with the water, and then stir into the vegetable mixture.

Bring to a boil and add the tofu. Stir thoroughly and immediately serve hot with steamed rice.

Serves 2 to 4.

Note: Tempeh can be used instead of tofu in this recipe. Tempeh is rather salty and stronger in flavor than tofu (use only 5 ounces). Cut into smaller cubes and fry until brown before adding to the sweet and sour mixture.

# CORN BREAD TAMALE PIE

PER SERVING: 379 CALORIES, 15.4 G PROTEIN, 58.9 G CARBOHYDRATE,
11.1 G FAT (1.9 G SATURATED), 1379.4 MG SODIUM, 9.6 G FIBER.

### Filling:

1 medium onion, chopped

2–3 cloves garlic, minced

½ cup green bell pepper, chopped (seeds and membrane removed)

½ cup red bell pepper, chopped (seeds and membrane removed)

2 medium zucchini cut into ½-inch cubes

1 eggplant, medium-sized, cubed

10 ounces firm tofu, drained and crumbled

10–12 mushrooms, sliced

1 cup tomato sauce or puree

1 cup chicken or vegetable stock

¼ teaspoon pepper

1 teaspoon salt

1 tablespoon chili powder

pinch of cayenne pepper or to taste

1 cup corn, fresh or frozen kernels

### Topping:

¾ cup cornmeal

1 tablespoon flour

1 tablespoon sugar

½ teaspoons salt

1½ teaspoons baking powder

1 egg, lightly beaten

⅓ cup soy milk*

1 tablespoon vegetable oil

1 teaspoon finely chopped jalapeño chile, seeds and membrane removed

*Vitasoy Creamy Original or other brand

Preheat oven to 400°F.

Sauté onion, garlic, red and green peppers, zucchini, eggplant, tofu, and mushrooms until tofu is lightly browned and onion is translucent. Add tomato sauce, stock, pepper, salt, chili powder, cayenne, and corn. Lower heat and simmer for about 5 minutes. Prepare topping: Mix the corn meal, flour, sugar, salt, and baking powder. Beat together egg, soy milk, and vegetable oil, and add to flour mixture. Add jalapeño and stir just to combine.

Place vegetable/tofu mixture in a buttered baking dish and spoon the corn bread topping on top. (Note: the topping may sink to the bottom, but will rise when baked.) Bake about 20-25 minutes until corn bread is nicely browned.

Serves 4-6.

*Recipe from* Healthy & Delicious Recipes, Vol. 1. *By permission of Vitasoy.*

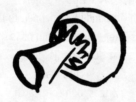

# STEWED BEAN CURD SKIN AND CLOUD EARS WITH PORK

PER SERVING: 370 CALORIES, 27.3 G PROTEIN, 7 G CARBOHYDRATE,
22.8 G FAT (4.8 G SATURATED), 717.4 MG SODIUM, .7 G FIBER.

¾ ounce (20 grams) cloud ears or tree ears (wood fungus)
3½ ounces (100 grams) bean curd skin (also called bean curd sticks or
bamboo yuba)
7 ounces pork country ribs (from the loin) or center-cut pork chops
1 tablespoon plus 1 teaspoon Chinese rice wine (Shao Hsing) or dry sherry
2 tablespoons plus 2 teaspoons dark soy sauce
2 tablespoons plus 2 teaspoons red fermented bean curd (can omit if
unavailable)
¼ teaspoon sugar
freshly ground black pepper, to taste
1 tablespoon plus 1 teaspoon cooking oil (soy, peanut, canola)
4 cloves garlic, diced
1¼ cups water
½ teaspoon cornstarch
fresh coriander (Chinese parsley, cilantro) leaves, to garnish

Soak the wood fungus in hot water and remove any debris.
Change the water if necessary. If fungus is not already shredded
when bought, cut it into small pieces after soaking for 30 minutes.

Break the bean curd skin into 1¾- to 2-inch lengths and soak
in hot water separately.

Trim pork of visible fat. Cut the meat into bite-size portions
and marinate with the wine, dark soy sauce, fermented bean curd,
sugar, and black pepper to taste. (Bones from the meat may be left
whole if they can't be cut. Include them in the stew as they contribute flavor and calcium.)

Heat the oil until it is fragrant in a heavy saucepan and add the
garlic. Sauté until aromatic, then add the marinated pork. Brown
the meat, turning it frequently.

Drain the wood fungus and bean curd skin, discarding the
water. Add the fungus and bean curd to the saucepan. Sauté for

5 minutes, then add 1 cup of water. Bring to a boil, reduce the heat slightly, and simmer for 40 minutes.

Mix the cornstarch with the remaining ¼ cup water and stir into the stew 5 minutes before the end of the cooking time.

Serve hot, garnished with the coriander leaf and accompanied by steamed rice.

Serves 4 to 6.

❖ ❖

Wood fungus is also known as cloud ear, wood ear, and tree ear. An albino form of this mushroom is called silver ear. Dehydrated packaged wood fungus can be bought from Asian food stores and some large supermarkets. It is available preshredded or whole, and it has to be soaked in hot water before use. It swells 5 to 6 times in size and resembles an ear after reconstituting; hence the common names. Wood fungus is reputed to possess anticoagulation properties that decrease the stickiness of platelets in the blood.

Bean curd skins, available from Asian groceries and some health food stores, are known as bean curd sticks or bamboo yuba in some countries. Protein content varies greatly among the various brands of this product.

Fermented red bean curd (a.k.a. "bean cheese") is available from Asian groceries. It has a rich, powerful flavor, similar to gorgonzola cheese. Once gotten used to, the flavor can be addictive.

❖ ❖

# STIR-FRIED TEMPEH
# AND VEGETABLES

PER SERVING: 172 CALORIES, 10.4 G PROTEIN, 20.7 G CARBOHYDRATE,
5.8 G FAT (.4 G SATURATED), 707.6 MG SODIUM, 3.8 G FIBER.

3½ ounces tempeh

2 teaspoons cornstarch

2 cloves garlic, diced

2 teaspoons cooking oil (soy, peanut, or canola)

1 medium carrot, cut into rings or julienned

3½ ounces baby corn (spears), halved lengthwise

⅓ cup broccoli, cut into small florets

¾ cup sugar snap peas, ends trimmed

2 tablespoons plus 1 teaspoon oyster sauce

1 tablespoon plus 1 teaspoon light soy sauce

¼ teaspoon salt

freshly ground black pepper, to taste

½ medium red bell pepper, cut into chunks

⅓ cup water

Cut the tempeh into slices ¼-inch thick, and then cut each slice into 3 pieces. Sprinkle 1½ teaspoons of the cornstarch over the tempeh pieces to coat them.

Sauté half of the garlic in 1 teaspoon of the soybean oil. Add the tempeh and sauté until brown on the surface, about 5 to 6 minutes. Add the carrot and stir-fry for 2 minutes before adding the baby corn.

Cook for 2 more minutes, and then add the broccoli, sugar snap peas, oyster sauce, soy sauce, salt, and pepper to taste. Stir for a minute, then add bell pepper. Sprinkle in some water if too dry.

Mix the remaining ½ teaspoon cornstarch with the remaining water and add to the vegetables. Stir well and cover for a minute before transferring to a serving plate or dish.

Serve with steamed rice or noodles.

Serves 3 to 4.

# TOFU CUTLET IN LETTUCE LEAVES WITH PRAWNS

PER SERVING: 439 CALORIES, 30.5 G PROTEIN, 11.7 G CARBOHYDRATE,
30.2 G FAT (4 G SATURATED), 654.3 MG SODIUM, 1.8 G FIBER.

3½ ounces fresh prawns, peeled and deveined
1 teaspoon light soy sauce
7 ounces ground pork (see Glossary)
1 tablespoon plus 1 teaspoon dark soy sauce
1 teaspoon oyster sauce
¾ ounce dried shiitake mushrooms
1 medium onion
⅔ cup (3½ ounces) water chestnuts (drained if canned, carefully peeled and
trimmed with a paring knife if fresh)
3½ ounces grilled tofu cutlet (p. 80)
12 lettuce leaves (iceberg is preferable)
2 tablespoons plus 2 teaspoons cooking oil (soy, peanut, canola)
1 teaspoon cornstarch
scant ¼ cup water or stock
¼ teaspoon salt
2 pinches of ground black pepper

Cut the shrimp into ¼-inch cubes, and then marinate in the light soy sauce.

Marinate the pork in the dark soy sauce and oyster sauce. (If dark soy is unavailable, use whatever soy is on hand and add a generous pinch of sugar.)

Soak the mushrooms in hot water and clean off the dirt before dicing. Dice the onion and water chestnuts, and cut the tofu into ¼-inch cubes. Rinse the lettuce leaves and trim into round shapes. Drain well.

Heat the oil in a wok. Sauté the onions for 2 minutes before adding the pork and mushrooms. Stir-fry for 5 minutes, and then add the water chestnuts and tofu.

Mix the cornstarch with the water, salt, and pepper. Add to the wok and stir through, and then add the shrimp and continue stirring until the shrimp are cooked, about 3 to 4 minutes.

When the mixture is nearly dry, spoon some of the mixture into each of the individual lettuce leaf rounds. Serve immediately.

Serves 4 to 6.

❖ ❖

This dish can be served as an entrée or appetizer, or as part of the main course with steamed rice and salads. Prawns may be omitted if desired.

❖ ❖

# SOYBEAN SPROUTS
# WITH GROUND PORK

PER SERVING: 153 CALORIES, 9.1 G PROTEIN, 8.3 G CARBOHYDRATE, 9.9 G FAT (2 G SATURATED), 471.1 MG SODIUM, 1.2 G FIBER.

13 ounces soybean sprouts
3½ ounces ground pork (see Glossary)
1 teaspoon dark soy sauce
1 tablespoon plus 1 teaspoon light soy sauce
1 tablespoon plus 1 teaspoon oyster sauce
1 teaspoon Chinese rice wine (Shao Hsing) or dry sherry
1 tablespoon plus 1 teaspoon cooking oil (soy, peanut, or canola)
2 cloves garlic, diced
½ cup water or chicken stock
¼ teaspoon salt
2 pinches of black pepper
1 teaspoon cornstarch
diced fresh red chile and/or green onion and/or coriander leaves,
to garnish

Wash the soybean sprouts and separate the white root from the yellow cotyledons (seed leaves), removing any stringy end roots. Chop up the cotyledons and drain the roots. Set aside.

Marinate the pork in the dark soy sauce, 1 teaspoon of the light soy sauce, 1 teaspoon of the oyster sauce, and the wine.

Heat 2 teaspoons of the soybean oil in a wok over high heat. Sauté half of the garlic until brown. Stir in the white soy roots and the remaining 3 teaspoons light soy sauce. Add half of the water and cook for 1 minute. Transfer to a serving plate, spreading over the plate evenly.

Reheat the wok and add the remaining 2 teaspoons of oil and the remaining garlic. Add the marinated pork and stir-fry for 3 minutes, before adding the yellow cotyledons from the soybean sprouts. Stir well, adding in the remaining 2 teaspoons of oyster sauce, salt, and pepper.

Cover and allow to cook for 2 minutes. Meanwhile, mix the cornstarch with the remaining water. Stir into the stir-fried pork, mixing well, and cook for further 1 to 2 minutes before transferring to the top of the cooked soy roots.

Serve garnished with red chiles and/or green onions and/or coriander leaves.

Serves 4.

**Note:** This dish goes well with salads and noodles or steamed rice.

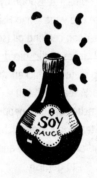

# SOYBEAN SPROUTS WITH SHREDDED BEEF

PER SERVING: 163 CALORIES, 12.1 G PROTEIN, 8.1 G CARBOHYDRATE, 8.8 G FAT (1 G SATURATED), 431.4 MG SODIUM, .8 G FIBER.

3½ ounces filet mignon, beef tenderloin, or sirloin strip (New York), cut against the grain into thin strips

¾-inch piece of fresh ginger, finely julienned

1 tablespoon plus 1 teaspoon light soy sauce

2 tablespoons oyster sauce

1 tablespoon plus 1 teaspoon Chinese rice wine (Shao Hsing) or dry sherry

pinch of ground black pepper

7 ounces soybean sprouts

1 tablespoon plus 1 teaspoon cooking oil (soy, peanut, or canola)

2 cloves garlic, diced

1 teaspoon cornstarch

scant ⅓ cup water or stock

Place the beef, ginger, soy sauce, ½ tablespoon of the oyster sauce, wine, and pepper in a bowl. Mix and set aside to marinate. Wash the soybean sprouts and remove unsightly tips or roots.

Heat ½ tablespoon of the oil in a wok over high heat. Add half the garlic and cook until just starting to brown. Add the soybean sprouts and stir-fry for a couple of minutes, then stir in the remaining oyster sauce. Cover the wok and continue cooking for 2 minutes.

Mix the cornstarch with half of the water. Add to the wok and continue to cook, uncovered, for a further 2 minutes. Transfer the soybean-sprout mixture to a serving plate.

Heat the remaining oil in the wok. Stir-fry the remaining garlic until light brown. Add the marinated beef.

Stir quickly for 2 minutes, and then add the remaining water. Allow to cook, covered, for a further minute.

Transfer the shredded beef to the top of the cooked soybean sprouts and serve immediately.

Serves 3 to 4.

**Note:** This dish goes well with steamed rice or noodles.

# SOYBEAN SPROUTS WITH SHRIMP

PER SERVING: 195 CALORIES, 19.2 G PROTEIN, 4.8 G CARBOHYDRATE,
10.7 G FAT (.4 G SATURATED), 473.9 MG SODIUM, .4 G FIBER.

7 ounces fresh shrimp (prawns), peeled and deveined
1 tablespoon plus 1 teaspoon light soy sauce
1 tablespoon plus 1 teaspoon oyster sauce (optional)
1 teaspoon Chinese rice wine or dry sherry
freshly ground black pepper, to taste
7 ounces soybean sprouts
2 tablespoons cooking oil (soy, peanut, or canola)
2 cloves garlic, chopped fine
¼ teaspoon salt
1 teaspoon cornstarch
2 tablespoons plus 2 teaspoons water
fresh coriander (Chinese parsley, cilantro) leaves, to garnish

Marinate the shrimp in the soy sauce, oyster sauce (if using),
wine, and pepper to taste for 10 minutes.

Wash the soybean sprouts and remove the tails if desired. Set
aside to drain. Heat the oil in a wok or frying pan, and then add
the garlic and stir-fry until fragrant. Add the shrimp and the marinade. Cook for 2 to 3 minutes, and then quickly remove the
shrimp from the wok and set aside on a plate.

Now add the soybean sprouts to the wok, tossing frequently
for about 5 minutes over high heat. Add the salt during cooking.

Return the shrimp to the wok and stir well. Mix the cornstarch into a paste with the water and stir into the wok.

When sauce is thick, transfer the wok's contents to a serving
plate and garnish with fresh coriander. Serve hot with boiled rice.

Serves 3 to 4.

❖ Soybean sprouts are rich in vitamin C, phytic acid, and phytoestrogens. The bright-yellow cotyledons contain most of the
nutrients found in the bean itself, and they are very crunchy in
texture and rather nutty in flavor.

# BAKED SOYBEANS IN EGGPLANT

PER SERVING: 280 CALORIES, 18.2 G PROTEIN, 24.5 G CARBOHYDRATE,
13.5 G FAT (4.1 G SATURATED), 142.4 MG SODIUM, 8.1 G FIBER.

1 large eggplant, about 10 to 11 ounces
1 teaspoon olive oil
1 small onion, diced
1 clove garlic, diced
2 ounces lean ground beef or lamb
3 tablespoons soybeans mixed with 1 tablespoon tomato paste and 1 tablespoon
water, or 4 tablespoons soybeans canned in tomato sauce (if available)
1 small tomato, diced
⅔ cup cauliflower, cut into small florets
salt and freshly ground black pepper, to taste
3 or 4 sweet basil leaves, shredded
2 tablespoons grated Parmesan cheese

Preheat the oven to 325°F.

Cut the eggplant lengthwise and carve out the inside of the eggplant to form the shape of a boat. Reserve the flesh for another use, such as a vegetable curry or, if very seedy, discard it.

Heat the oil in a saucepan over medium heat and sauté the onion and garlic until brown. Add the beef, soybeans, tomato, and cauliflower. Season to taste with salt and pepper. Cook for 2 minutes.

Place the eggplant skin side down in an ovenproof dish or casserole. Pack the meat filling into the hollowed-out eggplant. Sprinkle the basil and cheese over the top. Bake in the oven for 40 minutes.

Serve hot with boiled noodles and a green salad.

Serves 2.

Note: Vegetarians may substitute cooked white or brown rice or chopped walnuts for the meat in this recipe.

# STIR-FRIED RICE NOODLES

PER SERVING: 485 CALORIES, 15.1 G PROTEIN, 6.6 G CARBOHYDRATE,
14.9 G FAT (.6 G SATURATED), 1427 MG SODIUM, .6 G FIBER.

8 ounces rice noodles
2 green onions
2 cloves garlic
1 large egg
½ teaspoon salt
pinch of ground black pepper
2 tablespoons plus 2 teaspoons cooking oil (soybean, peanut, canola)
3½ ounces grilled or baked tofu cutlet, cut into strips (see p. 80)
3½ ounces peeled small shrimp (or cooked shredded chicken)
2 tablespoons plus 2 teaspoons oyster sauce
4 tablespoons light soy sauce
8 ounces bean sprouts, rinsed and drained

Soak the rice noodles in lukewarm water for 10 minutes. Separate the strands before draining. Dice the white part of the onion with the garlic; cut the green stems into 1¼-inch lengths. Set aside.

Beat the egg with the salt and pepper. Heat 1 teaspoon of the oil in a wok over medium heat. When the oil is hot, add the beaten egg and spread the egg over the bottom of the wok as if cooking a thin crêpe. When the egg is just cooked, remove from the pan—do not overcook the egg, as this will make it rubbery. Allow it to cool before cutting into ¾- to 1-inch strips. Set aside.

Heat the remaining oil in the wok and stir-fry diced garlic and spring onion until light brown. Add the tofu cutlet and chicken (if using). Stir-fry gently before adding the oyster sauce and 1 teaspoon of the light soy sauce. Add the rice noodles and the remaining soy sauce, and stir-fry over high heat, stirring constantly, for 7 to 8 minutes. Make a depression in the center of the rice noodles and add the bean sprouts. Season to taste with salt and pepper. Stir-fry for 4 to 5 minutes, adding the shrimp (if using) during the final two minutes. Add the cooked egg and green spring onion stems. Mix well and serve immediately.

Serves 4.

# STIR-FRIED CHINESE CABBAGE AND BEAN THREAD NOODLES

PER SERVING: 207 CALORIES, 7.1 G PROTEIN, 10.1 G CARBOHYDRATE,
14.4 G FAT (1.9 G SATURATED), 503.5 MG SODIUM, 1.8 G FIBER.

2 ounces bean thread noodles (cellophane vermicelli)
3½ ounces ground pork (see Glossary)
2 teaspoons Chinese rice wine (Shao Hsing) or dry sherry
2 tablespoons plus 2 teaspoons oyster sauce
1 tablespoon plus 1 teaspoon light soy sauce
freshly ground black pepper, to taste
½ small Chinese (Nappa) cabbage
2 tablespoons plus 2 teaspoons oil (soy, peanut, canola)
2 cloves garlic, diced
1 medium carrot, shredded
¼ teaspoon salt
1 teaspoon cornstarch
½ cup water

Soak the noodles in cold water for 20 minutes. Drain well and cut noodles into 4- to 6-inch lengths. Set aside.

Marinate the pork in the wine, 1 tablespoon of the oyster sauce, the soy sauce, and pepper to taste for 15 to 20 minutes.

Rinse the Chinese cabbage and cut into bite-size pieces about ½-inch wide. Drain well.

Heat the oil in a wok and stir-fry the garlic until fragrant. Immediately stir in the marinated pork. Stir-fry for 4 to 5 minutes.

Add the Chinese cabbage and stir-fry for 2 to 3 minutes. Add the carrot and noodles. Stir well and cook for a further 3 to 4 minutes. Add remaining oyster sauce and the salt.

Mix the cornstarch with the water and stir into the wok. Cook for 2 minutes, then serve immediately.

Serve with other stir-fried vegetables and steamed rice.

Serves 4 to 6.

❖ Bean thread noodles, available from the Asian section of many supermarkets, are made from mung bean flour and are rich in proteins and vitamin B. They also contains phytoestrogens. Bean threads can also be used in soups. When deep-fried (without soaking) they puff up and expand spectacularly, making a wonderful crisp topping for stir-fries. ❖

# MEDITERRANEAN SPINACH PASTA

PER SERVING: 396 CALORIES, 20.4 G PROTEIN, 14.1 G CARBOHYDRATE,
12.2 G FAT (1.4 G SATURATED), 284.6 MG SODIUM, 4.8 G FIBER.

1 tablespoon olive oil
14 ounces firm tofu, drained and cut into ¾-inch cubes
1 small onion, coarsely chopped
1 red bell pepper, trimmed and seeded, cut into 1-inch squares
2 medium zucchini, sliced ¼-inch thick
1 14½-ounce can no-salt-added cut tomatoes, undrained
8 black olives or green Spanish olives
1 package (about 9 ounces) fresh spinach pasta*

*Azumaya or other brand

Heat oil in a wide, non-stick skillet over medium-high heat.
Sauté tofu until lightly browned; remove from pan and set aside.
Add onion, bell pepper, and zucchini to pan; sauté 3 minutes.
Return tofu to pan; add tomatoes and olives. Cover and simmer
until vegetables are barely tender, 5 to 7 minutes. Keep warm.

Meanwhile cook spinach pasta following package directions;
drain and place in a serving bowl. Add sauce and toss. Serve
warm.

Serves 4.

*Recipe from* Delicious and Easy Recipes for Tofu and Pasta. *By permission
of Azumaya.*

# SESAME TOFU AND SPINACH PASTA

PER SERVING: 786 CALORIES, 36.3 G PROTEIN, 9.5 G CARBOHYDRATE,
21.7 G FAT (2.4 G SATURATED), 805.6 MG SODIUM, 8 G FIBER.

7 ounces extra-firm tofu, drained (or use baked tofu, page 80)
about 2 tablespoons light soy sauce, or as needed
4 teaspoons olive oil (divided)
4 teaspoons sesame seeds
12 asparagus spears, trimmed
1 yellow bell pepper, cut into strips
2 cloves garlic, minced
7 cherry tomatoes, cut into halves
2 tablespoons Asian chili sauce or chili oil (to taste)
1 package (about 9 ounces) fresh spinach pasta*

*Azumaya or other brand

Place raw tofu on a plate, and lay another plate on top of it.
Place a 28-ounce can of soup (or any similar weight) on the top
plate. Let the tofu stand under the weight for about an hour or
overnight in the refrigerator. This will make it very firm. (This step
may be omitted if using baked tofu.) When ready, cut tofu into
strips and toss in a small bowl with the soy sauce to cover all sides.

Meanwhile, bring salted water to a boil in a very large pot.
Add pasta and cook, following package directions.

Heat 2 teaspoons olive oil in a small non-stick skillet over
medium heat. Roll tofu in sesame seeds and add tofu to skillet.
Sauté, turning gently, until golden brown on all sides. Set aside off
the heat.

Heat remaining 2 teaspoons olive oil and garlic in wide non-
stick skillet over medium heat just until fragrant. Add asparagus
and yellow bell pepper and sauté for about 5 minutes, or until just
tender. Add cherry tomatoes to skillet and sauté for 2 minutes.
Toss spinach pasta, vegetables, tofu, and chili sauce/oil in medium
bowl and serve.

Serves 2.

*Recipe from* Delicious and Easy Recipes for Tofu and Pasta. *By permission
of Azumaya.*

# EASY VEGETABLE LASAGNA

PER SERVING: 513 CALORIES, 31.1 G PROTEIN, 58.3 G CARBOHYDRATE,
15.7 G FAT (7.5 G SATURATED), 280.9 MG SODIUM, 4.4 G FIBER.

1 tablespoon olive oil
8 green onions, chopped
1 cup sliced fresh mushrooms
1 clove garlic (or to taste), minced
1 48-ounce jar plain spaghetti sauce of choice
1 8-ounce package "no cooking required" lasagna noodles, or regular lasagna noodles
½ 10½-ounce package low-fat firm silken tofu
1 10-ounce package frozen chopped spinach, defrosted and drained
1 egg
½ teaspoon salt (or to taste)
¼ teaspoon pepper
½ teaspoon crumbled dried oregano leaves
1 tablespoon shredded fresh basil leaves, or ½ teaspoon crumbled dried basil
1 8-ounce ball of skim milk mozzarella, shredded
about ¼ cup (or to taste) grated Parmesan cheese (optional)

Preheat oven to 350°F. Spray a 9 × 13-inch baking dish with
non-stick vegetable oil. Sauté green onions and mushrooms in olive
oil over medium heat until mushrooms are browned. Add garlic
and stir briefly until translucent. Add spaghetti sauce and set aside.

Meanwhile, if using lasagna noodles that require precooking,
follow package directions for cooking, boiling for the minimum
time recommended. Drain immediately and rinse with cold running water until thoroughly cooled.

Combine tofu, spinach, egg, and seasonings and mix well. In
the baking dish, begin with a bottom layer of spaghetti sauce mixture, followed by noodles, tofu mixture, and more noodles, and
top with remaining sauce. Cover pan of lasagna with aluminum
foil. Bake for 45 minutes. Remove foil and scatter cheese on top of
lasagna. Bake uncovered an additional 15 minutes. Allow to stand
at room temperature for 10 minutes before serving.

Serves 8-10.

*Recipe courtesy of the Indiana Soybean Board.*

# TUNA SOY-MAC CASSEROLE

PER SERVING: 362 CALORIES, 31.9 G PROTEIN, 24.6 G CARBOHYDRATE,
14.8 G FAT (.8 G SATURATED), 909.6 MG SODIUM, 2.5 G FIBER.

7 ounces soy macaroni
1 tablespoon plus 1 teaspoon olive oil
2 medium onions
1 7-ounce can tuna, drained
10 ounces silken tofu
1½ cups water
½ teaspoon salt
½ teaspoon ground black pepper
1 teaspoon onion powder
1 tablespoon plus 1 teaspoon cornstarch
2 medium tomatoes, sliced
1¾ cups grated cheddar cheese or soy cheese

Preheat the oven to 350°F. Cook the pasta in a large saucepan of boiling water for 12 minutes or until al dente. Drain well.

Heat the oil in a large saucepan. Dice 1 onion and add to the pan. Sauté until fragrant, and then add the tuna.

Blend the tofu in ⅔ cup of the water. Add the tofu mixture, salt, pepper, and onion powder to the tuna mixture. Add ⅔ cup more of the water.

Mix the cornstarch with the remaining scant ¼ cup of water and stir into the tuna mixture to thicken the sauce.

Add the pasta and stir through. Cut the remaining onion into slices and line a casserole dish with them. Pour half of the pasta mixture into the dish, spreading out slightly to cover the bottom of the dish. Place the tomatoes in a layer on top of this, and then cover with the remaining pasta mixture. Sprinkle the cheese over the top.

Cover the dish with aluminum foil and bake in the oven for 20 minutes. Serve hot, accompanied by a garden salad.

Serves 4 to 6.

**Note:** Soy milk can be used instead of tofu in this dish. Reduce the amount of water to a scant ¼ cup and use 1¾ cups soy milk.

# Pancakes, Breads, and Muffins

Soy Pancakes

Banana Oat Pancakes

Crusty Soy Bread

Herb and Cheese Focaccia

Cherry Muffins

Apple Muffins

Banana Oatmeal Muffins

Sweet Potato Muffins

Little Lemon and Green Tea Muffins

Double Chocolate Muffins

# SOY PANCAKES

PER SERVING: 281 CALORIES, 9.3 G PROTEIN, 37.9 G CARBOHYDRATE,
10.5 G FAT (1.9 G SATURATED), 441.5 MG SODIUM, 1.8 G FIBER.

½ cup soy flour
1 cup all-purpose flour
½ teaspoon of salt
generous 1¼ teaspoon baking powder
1 large egg, beaten
2 tablespoons plus 2 teaspoons sugar
scant 1 cup soy milk
1 tablespoon plus 1 teaspoon cooking oil

Sift the soy flour, flour, salt, and baking powder twice. Make a well in the center of the dry ingredients and add the egg. Mix together with a spoon, gradually drawing in more of the flour from the sides as you go.

Add the sugar and soy milk, and mix until the batter is smooth.

Heat a frying pan or crêpe pan over medium to high heat. Grease with the oil. When hot, drop 2 tablespoons of batter for each pancake into the pan. Gently level the batter into a round shape using the back of a spoon.

When the pancakes are golden brown underneath, turn them over and cook the other side. Adjust the heat while cooking if necessary.

Serve with your favorite jam and freshly whipped cream.
Serves 4 to 6.

# BANANA OAT PANCAKES

PER PANCAKE: 75 CALORIES, 2.4 G PROTEIN, 13.1 G CARBOHYDRATE,
1.8 G FAT (.4 G SATURATED), 131.8 MG SODIUM, 1.1 G FIBER.

½ cup rolled oats
½ cup unbleached flour
¼ cup soy flour
1 tablespoon baking powder
1½ cup plain soy milk
2 bananas, thinly sliced

In a large bowl, combine the rolled oats, unbleached flour, soy flour, and baking powder. Add soy milk and blend with a few swift strokes. Fold in banana slices.

Heat a non-stick griddle or pan. Pour in 1/4 cup of the batter. Cook for about 2 minutes or until bubbles appear on the surface. Flip the pancake and cook for another minute or until heated through. Serve pancakes with maple syrup, fruit spread, or apple-sauce.

Yields 12 pancakes.

*Recipe courtesy of the Indiana Soybean Board.*

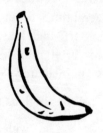

# CRUSTY SOY BREAD

PER SLICE: 111 CALORIES, 4 G PROTEIN, 20.6 G CARBOHYDRATE,
1.3 G FAT (.2 G SATURATED), 107.5 MG SODIUM, 1.1 G FIBER.

2½ cups bread flour
½ cup soy flour
½ cup soy milk
½ cup water
1 teaspoon salt
1 teaspoon sugar
1 package dry yeast

## Bread Machine Method:

Add ingredients to bread machine according to manufacturer's instructions. All ingredients should be at room temperature. Use the crusty bread setting for French bread.

## Conventional Method:

Mix dry ingredients together in a large mixing bowl. Gradually add liquids and knead the dough 2-3 minutes. Place the dough in bowl coated with a small amount of soy oil and turn once to coat dough. Cover with wax paper and a towel. Allow to rise in a warm place until doubled in size, about one hour. On a lightly floured surface, punch down several times to remove air bubbles and shape into a loaf. Place in 5 × 7-inch loaf pan. Cover and let rise 45 minutes. Bake at 350°F for 30-40 minutes. Remove from pan and cool on wire rack or serve immediately. Makes a 1½-pound loaf.

**Note:** This bread will not rise as high as traditional breads.

*Recipe from* It's Soy Easy...to Cook with Soy. *By permission of the Ohio Soybean Council.*

# HERB AND CHEESE FOCACCIA

PER SERVING: 223 CALORIES, 10.7 G PROTEIN, 34.6 G CARBOHYDRATE,
4.6 G FAT (1.7 G SATURATED), 449.7 MG SODIUM, 2.3 G FIBER.

1 package rapid-rise dry yeast
1 teaspoon sugar
¾ cup warm water (105° to 115°F)
¼ cup grated fresh Parmesan cheese
1 teaspoon seasoned salt
1 teaspoon garlic powder
1¼ teaspoon dried Italian seasonings
2 cups all-purpose flour
¼ cups soy flour
¼ cup additional fresh Parmesan cheese, coarsely grated or shredded

Dissolve yeast and sugar in warm water, stir to dissolve and set aside. Place ¼ cup Parmesan cheese, salt, garlic powder, Italian seasonings, and flours into a food processor and process 4-5 seconds. With processor running, slowly add yeast liquid through the feed tube until dough forms a ball, about 45 seconds. Dough will be slightly sticky. Place dough in a bowl coated with a small amount of soy oil and turn once to coat. Cover.

Let rise in a warm place until double in bulk, about 45 minutes. Punch down. Roll out on a floured surface into 12-inch circle and place on a pizza stone or pizza pan. Brush with remaining oil. Let rise 15 minutes.

Preheat oven to 375°F. Bake for 18-20 minutes. Sprinkle with the remaining cheese. Return to the oven for another 3 minutes or until cheese melts.

Serves 6.

**Focaccia Pizza:** Before baking, add toppings, such as sliced vegetables, mushrooms, grilled chicken, low-fat sausage, or soy-meat, and top with sliced skim-milk mozzarella and additional Parmesan cheese.

*Recipe from* It's Soy Easy…to Cook with Soy. *By permission of the Ohio Soybean Council.*

# CHERRY MUFFINS

PER MUFFIN: 189 CALORIES, 4.8 G PROTEIN, 31.8 G CARBOHYDRATE,
5.6 G FAT (.8 G SATURATED), 194 MG SODIUM, 2.1 G FIBER.

¾ cup soft brown sugar
1 tablespoon plus 1 teaspoon honey
¼ cup plus 1 tablespoon canola oil
2 large eggs, beaten
½ cup soy flour
1 cup whole wheat flour
generous 1½ teaspoons baking powder
½ teaspoon salt
⅔ cup soy milk
1 cup pitted cherries, halved

Preheat the oven to 350°F. Lightly grease muffin pans.

Mix the brown sugar, honey, and oil together in a large mixing bowl. Add the eggs to the mixture and stir strongly to combine thoroughly. Sift in the soy flour, whole wheat flour, baking powder, and salt and fold through well. Add the soy milk and stir until the batter is smooth. Fold in the cherries.

Spoon the batter into the prepared muffin pans and bake in the oven for about 20 minutes. Test with a wooden skewer after 17 minutes to check if cooked. When the skewer comes out clean, remove from the oven.

Allow the muffins to cool in the pan on a wire rack for a few minutes before turning out. They will keep for a few days if stored in an airtight container.

Makes 10 to 12 large or 28 to 30 small muffins.

❖ Canned pitted cherries can be used in this recipe. Cherries contain phytoestrogens. The batter may smell a little odd when wet because of the soy flour, but the smell invariably disappears with cooking. You can substitute an egg scrambler or 1 tablespoon soy milk for each egg in this recipe. ❖

# APPLE MUFFINS

PER MUFFIN: 208 CALORIES, 4.8 G PROTEIN, 33.6 G CARBOHYDRATE,
7.1 G FAT (.9 G SATURATED), 195.8 MG SODIUM, 2.3 G FIBER.

7 ounces apples, peeled and diced
¾ cup brown sugar
1 tablespoon plus 1 teaspoon honey
scant ⅓ cup canola oil
2 eggs, beaten
½ cup soy flour
1 cup whole wheat flour
generous 1½ teaspoon baking powder
½ teaspoon salt
⅔ cup soy milk
2 teaspoons ground cinnamon

Preheat the oven to 350 to 375°F. Grease 2 muffin pans.

Cook the apples in a microwave oven for 4 minutes. Set aside to cool.

Mix the brown sugar, honey, and oil together in a mixing bowl. Add the eggs and mix well. Sift the soy flour, wholemeal flour, baking powder, and salt into the bowl and combine thoroughly. Gradually mix in the soy milk and cinnamon. When the batter is smooth, fold in the cooled apples.

Spoon the batter into the prepared muffin pans and bake in the oven for 17 to 20 minutes, or until a metal skewer inserted into the center of a muffin comes out clean.

Allow the muffins to cool in the pan for a few minutes before turning out onto a wire rack.

Makes 10 to 12 large or 28 to 30 small muffins.

❖ Eggs can be omitted from this recipe and extra soy milk used in ❖
their place. Substitute 1 tablespoon plus 1 teaspoon soy milk for
each egg. The honey and soy flour give these muffins a very moist
texture. Do not be alarmed if the batter smells a little strange; this is
❖ due to the soy flour. The smell will disappear during baking. ❖

# BANANA OATMEAL MUFFINS

PER MUFFIN: 159 CALORIES, 4.4 G PROTEIN, 27.5 G CARBOHYDRATE,
4 G FAT (.6 G SATURATED), 250.5 MG SODIUM, 1.9 G FIBER.

1 cup old-fashioned oatmeal
¾ cup unbleached white flour
½ cup soy flour
½ cup sugar
1 tablespoon baking powder
½ teaspoon baking soda
½ teaspoon salt
3 medium very ripe bananas, peeled
1 cup unflavored yogurt or soy yogurt
2 tablespoons cooking oil
½ cup flaked or shredded coconut (optional)

Preheat oven to 375°F. Line 12 medium muffin cups with paper liners or spray bottoms with cooking spray.

In a food processor, process oatmeal until it resembles coarse flour, about 15 seconds. Add flours, sugar, baking powder, baking soda, and salt. Pulse a few times to combine. Transfer mixture to a large mixing bowl.

In processor, pulse bananas until coarsely mashed. Add yogurt and oil. Process until smooth.

Add wet ingredients to dry ingredients and stir by hand, quickly and lightly, until just mixed. (Batter will be thick.) Divide batter evenly between prepared muffin cups. Sprinkle with coconut, if desired. Bake for 20 to 25 minutes.

Makes 12 muffins.

*Recipe from Laura Nilsen, highlighted in* Veggie Life *(January 1999).*

# SWEET POTATO MUFFINS

PER MUFFIN: 139 CALORIES, 3.1 G PROTEIN, 30.1 G CARBOHYDRATE,
1 G FAT (.2 G SATURATED), 278.7 MG SODIUM, 2.1 G FIBER.

1 cup unbleached white flour
1 cup whole wheat flour
1 tablespoon baking powder
½ teaspoon baking soda
1 teaspoon grated orange zest
½ teaspoon salt
¼ teaspoon nutmeg
1 cup cooked sweet potatoes or yams
½ cup sugar
¼ cup orange juice
2 tablespoons vegetable juice
1 tablespoon molasses
1 cup plain soy milk
¼ cup finely chopped pecans (optional)
2 tablespoons brown sugar (optional)

Preheat oven to 375°F. Line 12 medium muffin cups with paper liners or spray bottoms with cooking spray.

In a food processor, combine flours, baking powder, baking soda, zest, salt, and nutmeg. Pulse a few times to mix. Transfer mixture to a large mixing bowl. In the processor, pulse sweet potato until mashed. Add sugar, orange juice, oil, and molasses. Process until mixed. Gradually add soy milk and process until smooth. Add wet ingredients to dry ingredients and stir by hand, quickly and lightly, until just mixed.

In a small bowl, mix together pecans and brown sugar, if using. Divide batter evenly between prepared muffin cups. Sprinkle with pecan mixture, if desired. (This will increase the calories and fat amounts from those shown.) Bake for 20 to 25 minutes.

Makes 12 muffins.

*Recipe from Laura Nilsen, highlighted in* Veggie Life *(January 1999).*

# LITTLE LEMON AND
# GREEN TEA MUFFINS

PER MUFFIN: 56 CALORIES, 1.6 G PROTEIN, 8.8 G CARBOHYDRATE,
1.6 G FAT (.2 G SATURATED), 107.1 MG SODIUM, .3 G FIBER.

1⅓ cups unbleached white flour
⅓ cup soy flour
⅓ cup sugar
1 tablespoon loose green tea, ground in a coffee or spice grinder
2 teaspoons baking powder
½ teaspoon baking soda
½ teaspoon salt
1 cup lemon-flavored yogurt or soy yogurt
2 tablespoons vegetable oil
½ teaspoon grated lemon zest
2 tablespoons mild honey (optional)
2 teaspoons lemon juice (optional)

Preheat oven to 375°F. Line 24 mini–muffin cups with paper liners or spray bottoms with cooking spray.

In a large bowl, whisk together flours, sugar, ground tea, baking powder, baking soda, and salt. In a small bowl, mix together yogurt, oil, and zest.

Add wet ingredients to dry ingredients and stir by hand, quickly and lightly, until just mixed.

Divide batter evenly between 24 prepared mini–muffin cups. Bake for 12 to 15 minutes.

If desired, prepare a honey-lemon glaze for the muffins by combining honey and lemon juice, heating for 10 seconds in a microwave and stirring until smooth. Drizzle glaze over hot muffins before removing from muffin pans.

Makes 24 muffins.

*Recipe from Laura Nilsen, highlighted in* Veggie Life *(January 1999).*

# DOUBLE CHOCOLATE MUFFINS

PER MUFFIN: 190 CALORIES, 4.1 G PROTEIN, 32.6 G CARBOHYDRATE,
4.2 G FAT (.8 G SATURATED), 393 MG SODIUM, 1.6 G FIBER.

1½ cups unbleached white flour
½ cup soy flour
1 cup brown sugar
⅓ cup unsweetened cocoa powder
1 tablespoon baking powder
1 teaspoon baking soda
1 teaspoon salt
1 cup chocolate soy milk
½ cup unflavored yogurt or soy yogurt
2 tablespoons vegetable oil
1 teaspoon vanilla
½ cup sliced almonds (optional)

Preheat oven to 375°F. Line 12 medium muffin cups with paper liners or spray bottoms with cooking spray.

In a food processor, combine flours, brown sugar, cocoa powder, baking powder, baking soda, and salt. Pulse a few times to mix. Transfer mixture to a large mixing bowl. Then, in the food processor, process soy milk, soy yogurt, oil, and vanilla until smooth. Add wet ingredients to dry ingredients and stir by hand, quickly and lightly, until just mixed.

Divide batter evenly between prepared muffin cups. Sprinkle with sliced almonds if desired. Bake for 20 to 25 minutes.

Makes 12 muffins.

*Recipe from Laura Nilsen, highlighted in* Veggie Life *(January 1999).*

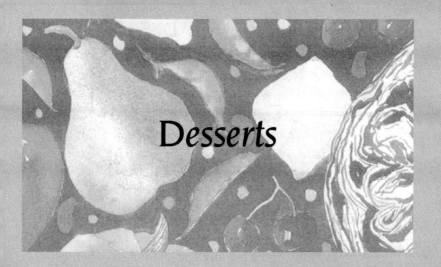

# Desserts

Strawberry Soy Dessert

Banana Berry Whip

Baked Honey Custard

Soy and Oatmeal Cookies

Banana-Topped Chocolate Silk Pie

"Heart Healthy" Pumpkin Pie

Soy Apple Cake

Soy Carrot Cake

Rich Cocoa Brownies

# STRAWBERRY SOY DESSERT

PER SERVING: 147 CALORIES, 4.6 G PROTEIN, 20.8 G CARBOHYDRATE, 4.4 G FAT (1 G SATURATED), 100.8 MG SODIUM, 1.9 G FIBER.

1 scant cup soy milk
1 cup strawberries, rinsed, hulled, and halved
4 teaspoons sugar or sweetener
2 teaspoons strawberry-flavored powdered milk*
2 teaspoons powdered gelatin
¼ cup hot water

*such as Nestle's Strawberry Quik

Pour the soy milk into a blender and add the strawberries. Add the sugar and Strawberry Quik, and blend for 30 seconds. Dissolve the gelatin in the hot water in a saucepan.

When the gelatin has dissolved completely, add the contents of the blender to the saucepan. Stir thoroughly.

Pour the mixture into 2 dessert bowls and allow to set in the refrigerator.

Serves 2.

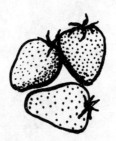

❖ Gelatin has a high protein content. Most strawberries are slightly sour in taste and therefore need more sweetening than other fruits. ❖

# BANANA BERRY WHIP

PER SERVING: 175 CALORIES, 4.8 G PROTEIN, 16.4 G CARBOHYDRATE,
2.4 G FAT (.1 G SATURATED), .7 MG SODIUM, 3.1 G FIBER.

¼ cup fresh or frozen raspberries
¼ cup fresh or frozen strawberries
1 peeled banana
4–6 ice cubes (omit if using frozen berries)
2 cups vanilla-flavored soy milk*

*Vitasoy Vanilla Delite or Light Vanilla or other brand

Blend all ingredients together in a blender until thick and
smooth.
Serves 2-3.

*Recipe from* Healthy and Delicious Recipes, Vol. 1. *By permission
of Vitasoy.*

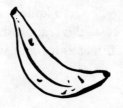

# BAKED HONEY CUSTARD

PER SERVING: 363 CALORIES, 10.7 G PROTEIN, 51.2 G CARBOHYDRATE,
13.6 G FAT (3.5 G SATURATED), 380.8 MG SODIUM, .1 G FIBER.

2 cups soy milk*
¼ cup honey
⅛ teaspoon salt
2 eggs, lightly beaten
1 teaspoon vanilla
cinnamon sugar
boiling water

*Vitasoy Creamy Original or other brand

Preheat oven to 300°F.

In a medium bowl combine soy milk, honey, and salt. Add eggs and stir in thoroughly. Pour mixture in custard cups or into a single 1-quart baking dish, such as a souffle dish. Set a larger pan on a rack in the center of the oven, place cups or baking dish in the pan, and pour in boiling water halfway up the cups or dish.

Bake for 20 minutes. Insert a knife between the edge of the custard and cup. The custard is ready if the knife comes out clean. The custard will grow firmer as it cools. When fully cooled, dust with cinnamon sugar.

Serves 4-6.

*Recipe from* Healthy and Delicious Recipes, Vol. 1. *By permission of Vitasoy.*

# SOY AND OATMEAL COOKIES

PER COOKIE: 93 CALORIES, 2.1 G PROTEIN, 12.5 G CARBOHYDRATE,
3.8 G FAT (2 G SATURATED), 54.2 MG SODIUM, 1.2 G FIBER.

½ cup butter, softened
¾ cup soft brown sugar
1 large egg
2 teaspoons vanilla extract
scant ½ cup low-fat soy milk
½ cup soy flour
½ cup plain (all-purpose) flour
½ teaspoon baking soda
2 teaspoons ground cinnamon
2½ cups quick-cooking rolled oats
1 teaspoon soybean oil, for oiling hands

Preheat the oven to 325°F. Grease 2 baking sheets.

Cream the butter and brown sugar together well. Beat in the egg and vanilla, and then the soy milk. Combine thoroughly.

Sift the soy flour, plain flour, baking soda, and cinnamon together. Add to the creamed mixture and mix well. Now add the rolled oats and mix until the dough is thoroughly combined.

Place a tablespoon of the dough into your oiled hands. Roll into a round ball before pressing the dough flat with the palms of your hands. Place the cookies on the baking sheets and bake in the oven for 20 minutes. Remove from the oven and slide the cookies off the baking sheets and onto a wire rack to cool.

Makes about 28 cookies.

**Note:** Five of these cookies contain approximately the same amount of phytoestrogens as 3½ fluid ounces of high-protein soy milk.

❖ Soy flour keeps better if stored in an airtight container in the refrigerator. Soy flour is heavier than wheat flour and retains a lot of moisture after baking. Rolled oats are very rich in fiber and also contain phytoestrogens.

# BANANA-TOPPED CHOCOLATE SILK PIE

PER SERVING: 440 CALORIES, 6.6 G PROTEIN, 57.1 G CARBOHYDRATE,
25 G FAT (10.6 G SATURATED), 140.6 MG SODIUM, 4 G FIBER.

12 ounces semisweet or dark chocolate
12 ounces soft silken tofu*
1 teaspoon pure vanilla extract
1 9-inch pie shell, baked
2 medium bananas
¼ cup melted semisweet chocolate for garnish
¼ cup chopped pistachios for garnish

*Azumaya or other brand

Chop the 12 ounces chocolate into small pieces. Melt the chocolate in the top of a double boiler over hot water, stirring often. While the chocolate is melting, puree the tofu in a food processor, stopping once or twice to scrape down the sides of the bowl with a rubber spatula. Add the chocolate and process until the tofu and chocolate are completely blended. Add the vanilla and pulse to blend.

Turn the chocolate mixture into the baked pie shell, spreading it with the spatula to fill the pie shell evenly. To set the filling, refrigerate the pie 60 minutes. Let the pie stand at room temperature for 15 minutes, uncovered, before serving. Cover the pie with thinly sliced bananas, then decorate it with drizzles of melted chocolate and chopped pistachios. This pie keeps 2 to 3 days in the refrigerator.

Serves 8-10.

*Recipe created by Dana Jacobi, adapted from* Delicious and Easy Recipes for Tofu and Pasta. *By permission of Azumaya.*

# "HEART HEALTHY" PUMPKIN PIE

PER SERVING: 269 CALORIES, 5.6 G PROTEIN, 41.6 G CARBOHYDRATE,
10.2 G FAT (2.4 G SATURATED), 241.5 MG SODIUM, 2.7 G FIBER.

pastry for a single-crust 9-inch pie
10 ounces firm tofu,* drained
½ cup white granulated sugar
¼ cup packed brown sugar
½ teaspoon salt
1 teaspoon ground cinnamon
½ teaspoon ground ginger
½ teaspoon ground nutmeg
¼ teaspoon ground cloves
1 teaspoon vanilla extract
1 large egg (optional)
1 16-ounce can pumpkin

*Azumaya or other brand

Preheat oven to 400°F.

Line a 9-inch pie pan with pastry; and prick bottom and sides with a fork. Partially bake crust for 10 minutes. If pie shell puffs during baking, remove from oven, again prick bottom and sides with fork, and return to oven. (Shell may also be baked filled with pie weights, dried beans, or rice to keep it from puffing.)

In a food processor, whirl tofu, white sugar, brown sugar, salt, cinnamon, ginger, nutmeg, cloves, vanilla, and egg until smooth. Push puree through a wire strainer placed over a large bowl. Add pumpkin to the puree; whisk together until evenly blended. Spoon filling into the pie shell, spreading it evenly. Return pie to 400°F oven for 15 minutes. Reduce oven heat to 350°F and continue to bake for 40 minutes longer.

Place on a rack and let cool to room temperature; then serve or refrigerate for up to 24 hours.

Serves 8.

*Recipe from* Delicious and Easy Recipes for Tofu and Pasta. *By permission of Azumaya.*

# SOY APPLE CAKE

PER SERVING: 476 CALORIES, 8 G PROTEIN, 67 G CARBOHYDRATE, 21.6 G FAT (3.2 G SATURATED), 515.9 MG SODIUM, 5 G FIBER.

4 medium green apples
1 teaspoon ground cinnamon
4 cloves
½ cup sugar
½ cup all-purpose flour
½ cup soy flour
¼ teaspoon baking soda
generous 1¼ teaspoons baking powder
½ teaspoon salt
scant ½ cup soy or canola oil
1 egg
scant ⅔ cup soy milk
⅓ cup shredded sweetened coconut

Preheat the oven to 325°F. Grease a deep, round 8- to 10-inch cake pan. Peel the apples and cut into thin slices. Add the cinnamon, cloves, and 1 tablespoon of the sugar, and cook for 4 minutes in a microwave oven. Set aside to cool.

Sift the flour, soy flour, baking soda, baking powder, and salt together. Beat the remaining sugar, oil, and egg together in a separate bowl. Add the sifted flours and fold through well, and then add the soy milk and stir until the batter is smooth.

Place the cooled apples in the bottom of the cake pan. Pick out the cloves and discard. Cover the apples with the cake batter and sprinkle the coconut evenly over the top.

Bake in the oven for 50 to 60 minutes, or until a skewer inserted into the center of the cake comes out clean. Cut the cake into 8 wedges while still in the pan and serve warm.

Serves 4 to 8.

**Note:** is recipe uses ingredients high in phytoestrogens and is extremely delicious. Canned cherries or seeded prunes can be used instead of fresh apples.

# SOY CARROT CAKE

PER SERVING: 246 CALORIES, 6.1 G PROTEIN, 36.9 G CARBOHYDRATE,
7.9 G FAT (1.1 G SATURATED), 389.5 MG SODIUM, 1.8 G FIBER.

½ cup soy flour
½ cup all purpose flour
1½ teaspoons baking powder
½ teaspoon baking soda
1½ teaspoons ground cinnamon
½ teaspoon salt
⅔ cup cooking oil
¾ cup sugar
2 eggs
½ cup pineapple pieces, chopped into smaller chunks
1 cup shredded carrots
¼ cup chopped pecans

Preheat the oven to 350°F. Grease a 10-inch round or 9-inch square cake pan.

Sift the soy flour, wheat flour, baking powder, baking soda, cinnamon, and salt together into a bowl.

Beat the oil, sugar, and eggs together in a separate bowl. Gradually add the sifted dry ingredients, stirring continuously, until everything is well incorporated.

Stir the pineapple, carrots, and pecans into the batter. Pour the batter into the prepared cake pan.

Bake in the oven for 50 to 60 minutes, or until a skewer inserted into the center of the cake comes out clean.

Allow to cool slightly in the pan before turning out onto a wire rack to cool. Store in an airtight container. This cake also freezes very well.

Serves 6 to 8.

**Cream Cheese Frosting:**

If you want to frost this cake, beat together ¼ cup butter, ½ teaspoon vanilla extract, and 4½ cups cream cheese. Slowly add 1½ cups confectioners' (icing) sugar to the creamed mixture, beating continuously, until you reach the desired consistency.

*Recipe adapted from an original by Mrs. Sherry Jordan.*

❖ ❖ Frosting is very sweet and high in calories, so simply leave the cake unfrosted if you are on a weight-reduction program. Cream cheese frosting is not suitable for freezing. ❖ ❖

# RICH COCOA BROWNIES

PER BROWNIE: 168 CALORIES, 3.6 G PROTEIN, 21.4 G CARBOHYDRATE,
7.9 G FAT (3.9 G SATURATED), 22.6 MG SODIUM, 3.1 G FIBER.

1 cup cocoa-flavored soy milk*

4 oz. unsalted butter

¼ cup honey

¼ cup maple syrup

1 teaspoon vanilla

⅓ cup cocoa powder

2½ cups whole wheat pastry flour

¼ teaspoon baking powder

¼ cup chopped nuts

*Vitasoy Rich Cocoa or Light Cocoa or other brand

Preheat oven to 375°F.

Melt the butter in a sauce pan and add the honey, syrup, vanilla, and cocoa powder. Remove from heat and stir in soy milk.

Sift together the flour and baking powder. Stir into the liquid cocoa mixture. Do not overmix. Fold in the nuts. Spread the batter into a greased and floured 8 × 8-inch baking pan. Bake in preheated oven for 35 minutes.

Let cool before cutting into 2-inch squares.

Makes 16 brownies.

*Recipe from* Healthy & Delicious Recipes, Vol. 1. *By permission of Vitasoy.*

# Health Glossary

(See p. 69 for Glossary of Ingredients.)

**Alzheimer's disease**  A degenerative condition affecting the brain and leading to dementia.

**antiangiogenic**  A substance that can prevent new blood vessels from forming, especially in a tumor. Rapidly growing tumors require a lot of nutrients for expansion and growth of their deviant cells, and nutrients are carried by the blood vessels. Thus, by stopping more blood vessels from growing around tumor sites, tumor growth is controlled.

**antibacterial**  A substance that can fight against germs.

**anticoagulant**  A substance that can thin or dissolve blood clots.

**antiestrogenic**  A substance that can oppose the effects of estrogens.

**antifungal**  A substance that can fight against fungus. A fungus belongs to the plant kingdom. An example of a fungus is candida.

**antihypertensive**  A substance that can control or lower blood pressure.

**anti-inflammatory**  A substance that can suppress or soothe inflamed parts of the body.

**antioxidants**  Chemicals that can prevent oxidation of food products. These chemicals prevent free oxygen radicals from harming the body; for example, they can prevent formation of cholesterol plaques within blood vessels. Examples of common antioxidants are vitamins C and E.

**antiviral**  A substance that can fight against viruses. An example of a virus is the common cold virus.

**benign**  Mild in character. In medicine, a benign tumor is not malignant.

**carcinogen**  Any substance that either promotes or initiates cancer.

**carotenemia**  Excessive carotene in the body due to overconsumption of carotene-containing foods. Usually manifests itself by an orange-yellow skin; most evident on the palms of the hands.

**cholesterol**  A fatlike substance produced by the liver or obtained from food. It is essential for the production of cell membranes, sex hormones, and vitamin D, among other things. High blood cholesterol levels are often associated with an increased risk of heart disease.

**coronary artery disease (CAD)**  A condition that may result in a heart attack. When the coronary arteries delivering blood to the heart become clogged with plaque, they can narrow and impair blood flow.

**coumestans**  Chemicals that are structurally related to isoflavones and have estrogenic effects. These are found in plant products such as alfalfa, clover, soybean sprouts, and other legume sprouts.

**daidzein**  Isoflavone found in soy that has been shown to have anticancer properties.

**DVT**  Deep venous thrombosis. This refers to clots in the deep veins inside the legs.

**estradiol**  Female hormone found in the blood of premenopausal women.

**estriol**  Female hormone found in the blood of pregnant women.

**estrone**  Female hormone found in the blood of menopausal women.

**fibroids**  Benign fleshy growths in the uterus (womb) that can cause problems with periods.

**fluid retention**  Can cause feelings of puffiness in the legs and fingers, and is often accompanied by a bloated tummy. It can result from a number of causes. Women may notice this problem around the time when they expect their periods to arrive.

**gastrointestinal**  Refers to the stomach, small bowel, and large bowel.

**genistein**  A chemical found in soy that has very strong estrogenic effects as compared to the other plant estrogens. It has a strong anticancer effect on the body.

**high-density lipoprotein (HDL)**  The body's major carrier of cholesterol to the liver for excretion in bile. Often referred to as "good cholesterol."

**HRT  Hormone replacement therapy**  This refers to giving humans hormones to treat a deficiency state. In the context of this book, it refers to estrogens, given either alone or in combination with a progesterone.

**isoflavones**  Compounds found in some plant products, which have estrogenic properties. These products' structure differs slightly from that of coumestans. Genistein and daidzein are examples of isoflavones.

**legumes** This food group includes fresh and dried beans, peas, lentils, and kidney beans.

**low-density lipoprotein (LDL)** Believed to take cholesterol from the blood and deposit it in the cells. Called "bad cholesterol" because studies indicate high levels of LDL enhance the risk of developing CAD (see above).

**menopause** Refers to a woman's last natural period. For most women, it is a retrospective label. A woman is said to have gone through menopause if she hasn't had a period in the preceding twelve months. If she still has a period every three to four months, or even every six months, she has not yet reached menopause.

**menses** Monthly periods.

**metabolism** Burning of energy to maintain cell function.

**nausea** A feeling of sickness in the stomach or belly, accompanied by an urge to throw up the stomach's contents.

**osteoporosis** Thinning of bone with loss of bone mineral density. It can result in easy fractures with or without minimal trauma.

**Pap smear** Sampling of cells from the cervix (mouth of the womb) to detect early cervical cancer.

**perimenopause** Years immediately preceding menopause (see above). Perimenopausal women may experience irregularity in their periods, accompanied by some menopausal symptoms such as hot flushes, mood changes, and sleeplessness.

**phytic acid** A chemical present in some plant products that can bind up metals such as zinc, calcium, iron, etc. If it is ingested in large quantities, a person may experience cramps at night.

**phytoestrogens** Naturally occurring compounds with estrogenic properties found in some plants. Phytoestrogens are similar in structure to human estrogens, but their effects are very weak compared to those of human estrogens.

**premenopause** Years of a woman's life before menopause.

**progesterone** The other female hormone produced by the ovaries. In general, progesterone has antiestrogenic effects.

**protease inhibitor** A chemical that blocks the action of specific enzymes thought to be responsible in the formation or growth of tumors.

**tempeh** A fermented soybean product that has a meaty, nutty taste. It is rich in proteins, iron, calcium, and B-group vitamins.

**tofu** Soybean curd made from concentrated soy milk, with a coagulant added to set the mixture. Weight for weight, tofu is not as concentrated in nutrients as tempeh.

**transit time** Time taken for the passage of a food item. In the context of this book, refers to the time the item takes to pass through the digestive system.

**triglycerides** A type of fat that is manufactured by the liver and obtained from dietary fat. Triglycerides circulate in the bloodstream and are either used for energy or stored in body tissues as fat. Elevated levels are common in coronary artery disease.

# Resources

**Information on Soy Products**

The United Soybean Board
Toll-free phone: 800-825-5769
www.soyfood.com

**Ordering Soy Products**

BodyLogic Soy and Flaxseed products (Cereal Crumble, Rice Snackle Bars, Oy-Soy Trail Mix, Soylent Beans & Greens Topping):
8895 Towne Centre Drive, #105
San Diego, CA 92122
Toll-free phone and fax: 888-594-2232
www.body-logic.com

Revival Soy Shake (used at Johns Hopkins to treat women at high risk for breast cancer):
Toll-free phone for information: 800-700-8687
Toll-free phone for ordering: 800-700-1560
www.revivalsoy.com

Take Care Soy Drink (used in 1996 Wake Forrest Study of menopausal women):
Call Nutritious Foods
Toll-free phone: 800-445-3350

Mori-nu Tofu (aseptically packaged tofu; it can be shipped anywhere in the United States):
Toll-free phone: 800-NOW-TOFU

**Ordering Natural Progesterone**

Progest (Transitions for Health):
Toll-free phone: 800-888-6814

FemGest (Women's Wisdom Nutritional):
Toll-free phone: 800-705-5559

## Mail Order Sources For Ingredients

Haig's, 642 Clement St., San Francisco, CA 94118. (415) 752-6283. Indian and Southeast Asian foodstuffs and spices. No catalog, but write or phone for price quotes.

Penzeys, Ltd. Spices and Seasonings, P.O.Box 933, Muskego, WI 53150. (414) 679-7207. Internet: www.penzeys.com. Complete line of dried spices including Chinese Five Spice blend, Indian Garam Masala blend, dried lemongrass, star anise, curry powders.

Ratto's, 821 Washington Ave., Oakland, CA 94607. (510) 832-6503. International foods and spices, including Indian and Asian products.

Richters Herb Catalog, Goodwood, Ontario, Canada LOC 1A0. (905) 640-6677. Internet: www.Richters.com. Major source of herb seeds and live plants, including dried herbs of many types. Source for licorice root (dried roots; seeds), Dong Quai (live plants or seeds), lemongrass (live plants or powdered).

Uwajimaya, P.O. Box 3003, Seattle, WA 98114 (206) 624-6248. Japanese, Chinese, and Korean food products and equipment. Free catalog.

# References

Adlercreutz, H. 1996. Phytoestrogens from biochemistry to prevention of cancer and other diseases. Eighth International Congress on the Menopause Symposium, Sydney, Australia.

Adlercreutz, H., et al. 1992. Dietary phyto-oestrogens and menopause in Japan. *The Lancet* 339:1233

Albertazzi, Paola, et al. 1998. The effect of dietary soy supplementation on hot flushes. *Obstetrics & Gynecology* 91(1):6–11.

Anderson, J. J. B., and S. C. Garner. 1997. The effects of phytoestrogens on bone. *Nutrition Research* 17:1617–32.

Anderson, J. W., et al. 1995. Meta-analysis of the effects of soy protein intake on serum lipids. *New England Journal of Medicine* 333:276–82.

Baird, D. D., et al. 1995. Dietary intervention study to assess estrogenicity of dietary soy among postmenopausal women. *Journal of Clinical Endocrinology and Metabolism* 8:1685–90.

Bierenbaum, Marvin, et al. 1994. Reducing atherogenic risk in hyper-lipemic humans with flax seed supplementation: a preliminary report. *American College of Nutrition* 12(5):501–4.

Black, C. 1994. Menopause: the alternative way. *Australian Women's Research Centre* 1:62–80.

Boulet, M. J. 1994. Climacteric and menopause in seven south-east Asian countries. *Maturitas* 19:157–76.

Bungay, T., et al. 1980. Study of symptoms in middle life with special reference to the menopause. *British Medical Journal* 281:181–3.

Caroll, K. K. 1991, Review of clinical studies on cholesterol-lowering response to soy protein. *Journal of the American Dietary Association* 91:820.

Carper, J. 1993. *Food: Your Miracle Medicine.* New York: HarperCollins Publishers.

Cashel, K., R. English, and J. Lewis. 1989. *Composition of Foods.* Australia: Australian Government Publishing Service.

Cassidy, A., et al. 1994. Biological effects of a diet of soy protein rich in isoflavones on the menstrual cycle of premenopausal women. *American Journal of Clinical Nutrition* 60:333–40.

Colditz, Graham, et al. 1995. The use of estrogens and progestins and the risk of breast cancer in postmenopausal women. *New England Journal of Medicine* 332:1589–93.

Cunnane, Stephen C., et al. 1993. High alpha-linolenic acid flaxseed (Linum usitatissimum): some nutritional properties in humans. *British Journal of Nutrition* 69:443–53.

————April 11, 1995. Current concepts in the early detection of breast cancer. Third Annual Oncology Conference: American Cancer Society.

————1995. Nutritional attributes of traditional flaxseed in healthy young adults. *American Journal of Clinical Nutrition* 61:62–8.

Dalais, F. S., et al. 1996. The effects of phytoestrogens in postmenopausal women. Eighth International Congress on the Menopause Symposium, Sydney, Australia.

Dennerstein, L., et al. 1993. Menopausal symptoms in Australian women. *Medical Journal of Australia* 159:232–6.

Draper, C. R., et al. 1997. Phytoestrogens reduce bone loss and bone resorption in oophorectomized rats. *Journal of Nutrition* 127(9): 1795–9.

Dwyer, Johanna, et al. 1994. Tofu and soy drinks contain phytoestrogens. *Journal of the American Dietary Association* 94:739–43.

Eden, J. A. 1992. Oestrogen and the breast. The management of the menopausal woman with breast cancer. *Medical Journal of Australia* 157:247–9.

Eden, J. A., et al. 1996. A controlled trial of isoflavones for menopausal symptoms. Eighth International Congress on the Menopause Symposium, Sydney, Australia.

Edington, R. F., et al. 1980. Clonidine (Dixarit) for menopausal flushing. *Canadian Medical Association Journal* 123:23–6.

Erdman, J. W., and S. M. Potter. 1997. Soy and bone health. *Soy Connect* 5:1.

Fraser, Gary E. 1994. Diet and coronary heart disease: beyond dietary fats and low-density-lipoprotein cholesterol. *American Journal of Clinical Nutrition* 59 (suppl.):1117S–23S.

Gaddi, Antonio, et al. 1991. Dietary treatment for familian hypercholesterolemia—differential effects of dietary soy protein according to the apolipoprotein E phenotypes. *American Journal of Clinical Nutrition* 53:1191–6.

Goldin, B. R. 1994. Nonsteroidal estrogens and estrogen antagonists: mechanisms of action and health implications. *Journal of the National Cancer Institute* 86:174.

Goodman, Marc, et al. 1997. Association of soy and fiber consumption with the risk of endometrial cancer. *American Journal of Epidemiology* 146:294–306.

Greenstein, J., et al. 1996. Risk of breast cancer associated with intake of specific foods and food groups. *American Journal of Epidemiology* 143(11):S36.

Griffiths, K. 1996. Epidemiology of phytoestrogens, cancer and other diseases. Eighth International Congress on the Menopause Symposium, Sydney, Australia.

Hasler, Clare, and Susan Calvert Finn. 1998. Soy: just a hill of beans? *Journal of Women's Health* 7(5):519–23.

Herman, C., et al. 1995. Soybean phytoestrogen intake and cancer risk. *Journal of Nutrition* 125:757S–70S.

Hughes, C. J. 1996. Phytoestrogens. Eighth International Congress on the Menopause Symposium, Sydney, Australia.

Hully, Stephen, et al. 1998. Randomized trial of estrogen plus progestin for secondary prevention of coronary heart disease in post-menopausal women. Journal of the American Medical Association 280(7):605–13.

Hutchins, Andrea, et al. 1995. Vegetables, fruits, and legumes: effect on urinary isoflavonoid phytoestrogen and lignan excretion. *Journal of the American Dietary Association* 95:769–74.

Ingram, David, et al. 1994. Just the flax, Ma'am: researchers testing linseed. *Journal of the National Cancer Institute* 86:1746–7.

———1997. Case-control study of phyto-oestrogens and breast cancer. *The Lancet* 350:990–4.

Knight, D. C., and J. Eden. 1995. Phytoestrogens: a short review. *Maturitus* 22:167–75.

Knight, D. C., et al. 1996. A review of the clinical effects of phytoestrogens. *Obstetrics & Gynecology* 87:897–904.

Lampe, Johanna, et al. 1994. Urinary lignan and isoflavonoid excretion in premenopausal women consuming flaxseed powder. *American Journal of Clinical Nutrition* 60:122–8.

Lee, H. P., et al. 1991. Dietary effects on breast-cancer risks in Singapore. *The Lancet* 337:1197–200.

Little, B. 1986. *The Complete Book of Herbs and Spices*. New South Wales, Australia: Reed Books.

Llewellyn-Jones, D., and S. Abrahams. 1988. *Menopause*. Victoria, Australia: Ashwood House/Penguin Books, 65–75.

Louria, D. B., et al. 1985. Onion extract in treatment of hypertension and hyperlipidemia: a preliminary communication. *Current Therapeutic Research* 37:127–31.

Messina, Mark, and Stephen Barnes. 1991. The role of soy products in reducing risk of cancer. *Journal of the National Cancer Institute* 83(8):541–6.

Messina, Mark, et al. 1997. Phyto-oestrogens and breast cancer. *The Lancet* 350:971–2.

Murkies, A. L., et al. 1995. Dietary flour supplementation decreases post-menopausal hot flushes: effect of soy and wheat. *Maturitus* 21: 189–95.

National Health and Medical Research Council. 1992. *Dietary Guidelines for Australians*. Australia: Australian Government Publishing Service.

Potter, S. M. 1995. Overview of proposed mechanisms for the hypocho-lesterolemic effect of soy. *Journal of Nutrition* 125:606S.

Prince, R. 1993. The calcium controversy revisited: implications of new data. *Medical Journal of Australia* 159:404–6.

Riggs, B. L., and I. J. Melton. 1992. The prevention and treatment of osteoporosis. *New England Journal of Medicine* 327(9):602–27.

Sack, M. N., et al. 1994. Oestrogen and inhibition of oxidation of low-density lipoproteins in postmenopausal women. *Lancet* 343:269–70.

Saltman, D. 1994. *In Transition: A Guide to Menopause*. New South Wales, Australia: Choice Books.

Sojka, J. E., and C. M. Weaver. 1995. Magnesium Supplementation and Osteoporosis. *Nutrition Reviews* 53(3):71–4.

Stanton, R. 1989. *The Complete Book of Food and Nutrition*. Sydney, Australia: Simon & Schuster.

Stuart, M. 1982. *The Color Dictionary of Herbs and Herbalism*. London: Orbis Publishing.

Van Schaick, S. 1993. Symptomatic treatment of hot flushes. *Therapeutics Update* 61–5.

Vines, G. 1994. Cancer: is soy the solution? *New Scientist* July:14–5.

Wilcox, G. 1996. Effect of soy on menopausal symptoms. Eighth International Congress on the Menopause Symposium, Sydney, Australia.

Wilcox, G., et al. 1990. Oestrogenic effects of plant foods in post-menopausal women. *British Medical Journal* 30:905–6.

Wolk, Alicja, et al. 1998. A prospective study of association of monoun-saturated fat and other types of fat with risk of breast cancer. *Archives of Internal Medicines* 158:41–5.

# Appendix

A simplified diagram showing the phytoestrogens that are currently known to be important to humans

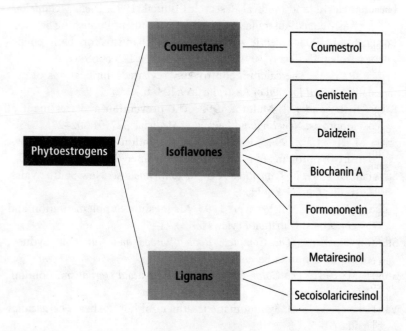

**Note:** Other, much less important phytoestrogens are omitted from the above diagram.

# Index

alcohol, 27, 41, 58; and breast cancer, 31
alfalfa, x, 17
alfalfa sprouts, 88
almonds, 41
alpha linoleic acid, 35
Alzheimer's disease, 12, 13, 198
amenorrhea, 55
anise seed, 17
antiangiogenic, 198
antibiotics, 55
antioxidants, 3, 19, 33, 36, 198
anxiety,10
appetizers, 81–91
Apple and Potato Salad, 108
Apple Muffins, 181
apples, 17; recipes with, 98, 108, 194
arginine, 33
Asian Chili Sauce, 133, 135
Asian diet, 18, 20
Asian women, 16
Asian-Style Chicken Stock, 77
atherosclerosis, 33

Baba Ghannouj, 83
backache,10
bacteria, 23, 28
Baked Honey Custard, 190
Baked Soybeans in Eggplant, 167
Banana Berry Whip, 189
Banana Oat Pancakes, 177
Banana Oatmeal Muffins, 182
bananas, recipes with, 89, 177, 182, 189, 192
Banana-Topped Chocolate Silk Pie, 192
barley, 17
basic recipes, 75–80
bean curd (see tofu)
Bean Salad, 105
Bean Sprouts in Fish Sauce, 125
bean thread noodles, 169–170
beans (see also chickpeas, legumes), 17, 35, 42

beef, recipes with, 149–150, 165
beets, 17
berries, recipes with, 188–189
beta carotene, 36, 90
biochanin A, 18
bioflavenoids, 23–24
black cohosh, 17
black-eyed peas, 17
bleeding, vaginal, 13
blood sugar, 33
bok choy, 17, 30
bone, 12; density, 3, 19; baseline test, 58; strengthening, 2
bone loss (see also osteoporosis), 38–42
boron, 24, 42
breads, 178–179
breakfast, 61
breast cancer, ix, 2, 3, 13, 18; and diet, 26–31
breast self-exams, 59
breast soreness, 13, 55
broccoli, 17, 30
brownies, 197
brussels sprouts, 30
B-vitamins, 24, 36–37, 45, 47, 51

cabbage, 17, 30
caffeine, 24, 55, 58; and bone loss, 41
calcium, 24, 41, 45, 47, 51; daily requirement, 57
cancers, 18; breast, ix, 2, 3, 13, 18, 26–31; colon, 3, 18; endometrial, 3; hormone-dependent, 13, 14, 26; prostate, 3, 18; uterine, 14
canola oil, 17, 34, 70
Cantaloupe Soy Milk Shake, 90
cantaloupes, 24
carbohydrates, 41
carotenemia, 55, 198
carrot cake, 195
carrots, recipes with, 101, 195
cauliflower, 30
celiac disease, 48

cereals, 17, 20
Cheesy Scalloped Potatoes, 126
cherries, 17, 24; recipes with, 180
Cherry Muffins, 180
chicken, daily servings, 56
chicken, recipes with, 136–142
Chicken Breasts with Chipotle Sauce, 141–142
chicken stock, 77
Chickpea Dip (Hummus), 82
Chickpea Salad, 104
chickpeas, 15, 17, 70, 119; cooking, 76; recipes with, 82, 104, 118, 120
chili sauce, 70
chipotle chile, 141–142
cholesterol, 2, 19, 32, 198
cinnamon, 137
citrus fruits, 24
cloud ears (wood fungus), 158–159
clover, ix, 15
cloves, 17
cod liver oil, 29
colon cancer, 3, 18
concentration, loss of, 11
conversion table, 67
Cooked Dried Chickpeas, 76
Cooked Dried Soybeans, 76
cookies, 191
copper, 42
Corn Bread Tamale Pie, 156–157
corn, 17; recipes with, 95
corn oil, 17
coronary artery disease, 199
coumestans, x, 15, 88, 199
Cream Cheese Frosting, 196
Creamy Basil Dressing, 117
Creamy Corn Soup, 95
Creamy Poppy Seed Dressing, 115
Creamy Potato Soup, 100
Creamy Pumpkin Soup, 98
Creamy Tomato Soup, 97
cruciferous vegetables, 30–31

Crusty Soy Bread, 178
cucumbers, 17
Curried Carrot Soup, 101
Curried Chickpeas,
    118–119
Curried Tofu and
    Vegetables, 146
custard, 190

daidzein, 18, 27, 39, 199
dashi, 71, 94
Deep Fried Tofu, 79
deep venous thrombosis,
    199
defatted soy flour, 48, 66
depression, 10
desserts, 187–197
diet, changing, 60–64
diet and breast cancer, 26–31
dinner, 61
dong quai, 15, 17
dosages, phytoestrogens, 4
Double Chocolate Muffins,
    185

Easy Vegetable Lasagna,
    173
edamame (see also soy-
    beans), 45
eggplant, recipes with, 83,
    167
eggs, 181
embolism, 13, 14
endometrial cancer, 3
endometriosis, 13
estradiol, ix, 27, 199;
    sources of, 108, 122
estriol, 199
estrogen-based cancers, 26
estrogens, ix, 10; level, 16;
    overexposure, 26; recep-
    tors, 15, recommended
    daily allowance, 54
estrone, 199; sources of, 108
exercise, 42, 57

fajitas, vegetable, 144
fat, body, 30
fat, dietary, 27, 28–29; serv-
    ings of, 57
fatigue, 11
fats, saturated, 29
fennel, 17, 138
Festive Vegetable Fajita
    Wraps, 144
fiber, dietary, 23, 29–30;
    daily servings, 56

fiber, soluble, 34–35
fibroids, uterine, 13, 199
fish, 29; daily servings, 56;
    recipes with, 139, 153
fish sauce, 107
flatulence, 5
flaxseed, x, 15, 24, 27, 35–36
flaxseed oil, 17
fluid retention, 13, 199
focaccia, 179
formononetin, 18
Fragrant Soy Sauce, 132,
    134
free radicals, 19
Fried Rice, 127–128
fruits, 17, 28; daily serv-
    ings, 56; recipe with, 91
fungus, wood, 158–159

Gado Gado, 130–131
garam masala, 70; recipe, 78
garbanzo beans (see
    chickpeas)
garlic, 17, 37
gelatin, 188
genistein, 18, 19–20, 27,
    33, 39, 199
ginger, 17, 140
ginseng, panax, 15
glucosinolates, 30
glycine, 33
grains, 17, 28, 35; whole,
    daily servings, 56
grapes, 17, 24
Greek Soybean Salad, 111
Greek Tofu Salad, 110
green beans, 17; nutrition
    content of, 122, 131;
    recipes with, 121
green pepper, 17, 24
Green Soybean Salad, 111
green tea, 38; recipe with,
    184
Grilled or Broiled Tofu
    Cutlet, 80
Grilled Soy Cheese
    Sandwiches, 88

hair, facial, 10
headaches, 10, 13
health guidelines, 56
Healthy Caesar Salad
    Dressing, 116
Healthy Chili, 145
heart disease, 2, 13, 31–
    39; and hormone

replacement therapy,
    31–32; and soy, 32–33
"Heart Healthy" Pumpkin
    Pie, 193
heart healthy strategies,
    34–38
Herb and Cheese Focaccia,
    179
herring, 29
Hoisin Sauce, 133, 135
homocysteine, 36–37
honey, 190
hops, 17
hormone modulation, 15
hormone replacement ther-
    apy, 1, 12–14, 199; and
    bone loss, 38–39; bene-
    fits, 12–13; risks, 14;
    side effects, 13
hormone-dependent
    diseases, ix
hot flashes, x, 2, 11, 19
Hot Pot (Steamboat),
    132–136
Hummus, 82
Hunanese Tofu Beef,
    149–150
hypertension, 2, 19

incontinence, 11
indole 3-carbinol, 30
insomnia, 10
intercourse, painful, 10
Ipriflavone, 19–20
iron, 47, 51
irritability, 10
isoflavones, 2, 15, 18, 20,
    26, 33, 199; sources of,
    41, 44
isoflavonoids, x
isolated soy protein, 61

Japanese diet, 21
joint aches, 11

kale, 30
ketjap manis, 71

lasagna, 173
lecithin, 50
legumes, 17, 20, 200; daily
    servings, 56
lentils, 17; recipes with, 85,
    99
Lentil-Vegetable Soup, 99
libido, loss of 11
licorice, 17

licorice root, 137
lignans, x, 15, 27–28, 88
Lime and Fish sauce, 133, 134
linoleic acid, 44, 50
Little Lemon and Green Tea Muffins, 184
liver disease, 13
low density lipoprotein, 19
low-fat diet, 24, 34
lunch, 61

mackerel, 29
magnesium, 41–42; daily requirement, 57
main courses, 129–174
mammograms, 58
manganese, 42
mayonnaise, tofu (recipe), 114
meat, daily servings, 56
Mediterranean Spinach Pasta, 171
memory, 11
men and estrogen diet, 59
menopause, ix, 1; definition of, 11, 200; symptoms of, 10–12
miso, 46, 71; nutritional content, 62; recipe with, 94
Miso Soup, 94
monounsaturated oils, 34
mood swings, 11, 12
MSG, 72, 113
muffins, 180–186
mung bean sprouts, 17; recipe with, 125
mung beans, 170
muscle aches, 11
mushrooms, 17
Mutabbal (Baba Ghannouj), 83

nausea, 13
navy beans, 17
night sweats, 21
nuts, 24, 42

oats, 17; recipe with, 177
oils, 24; cooking, 70
olive oil, 17, 34, 70
olives, 17
omega-3 fatty acids, 28, 29, 34, 35, 44, 50
omega-6 fatty acid, 44, 50
onions, 37

osteoporosis, 12, 13, 38–42, 200
ovaries,10
oyster sauce, 72, 132, 134, 148

pancakes, 174–177
papaya, 17
pasta and noodle recipes, 168–174
peanut oil, 70
peanut sauce, 132, 135
peanuts, 17
pears, 17
peas, 17
peppers, green, 17
perimenopause (definition), 1, 11, 59, 200
phytates, 33
phytic acid, 200; source of, 166
phytoestrogens, 2, 15; and bone loss, 39–40; and cancer, 26–31; and menopausal symptoms, 14–15; definition, ix–x, 200; factors affecting, 22–23; function of, 16, 18; sources of, 138, 140, 166, 170
phytohormones, 15
pick-me-ups, 81–91
Plain Baked Tofu Cutlet, 80
plant estrogens (see phytoestrogens)
Plum Sauce, 133, 135
plums, 17
Poached Spiced Chicken, 136–137
polyphenols, 38
polyunsaturated oils, 29, 34
pomegranates, 17, 108
pork, ground, 71; recipe with, 86, 163–164
potassium, 51
potatoes, 17; recipes with, 98, 100, 108, 126
prawns, recipe with, 123, 161, 166
premenopause, 26, 200
progesterone, 3, 38–39, 200
progestins, 3
prostate cancer, 3, 18
protein and soy, 44, 51
prunes, 17
pumpkins, 17; recipe with, 98, 193

pumpkinseed, 17

radishes, 30
raloxifene, 27
rapeseed oil, 17
red beans, 17
red clover, 3, 17
rhubarb, 17
rice, 17
Rich Cocoa Brownies, 197
rose hips, 24
rye, 15, 17

sage, 17, 138
salad dressings, 113–117
salads, 103–112
salicylates, foods with, 55
salmon, 29
salt, 58
saponins, 33
Satay Peanut Sauce, 132
saturated fats, 34
seaweed, 17
seeds, 17, 24
Sesame Chicken Fillet, 130
sesame oil, 17
sesame seeds, 17, 140
Sesame Tofu and Spinach Pasta, 172
sexual drive, lack of, 11
shrimp (see prawns)
side dishes, 118–128
skin, dry, 10; itchy, 11
sleep, 58
smoking, 58; and bone loss, 41
smoothies, 91
snacks, 81–91
snow peas, recipe with, 123
soda drinks and bone loss, 41, 58
sodium, 47, 48
soups, 93–101
soy, 2, 15, 44–52; adding to diet, 60–64; and bone loss, 39–40; and cancer, x, 26–31; and heart disease, 32–33; and hot flashes, 20–21; minimum daily requirement, 20–22
Soy and Oatmeal Cookies, 191
Soy Apple Cake, 194
Soy Carrot Cake, 195–196
soy cheeses, 51; recipe with, 88

soy drinks, nutritional content, 63
soy flour, 20, 48; defatted, 66; recipes with, 176, 178, 191; storing, 191
soy foods, daily servings, 56; nutritional content, 62–64
soy grits, 51
Soy Macaroni Salad, 109
soy milk, 45–46, 91; low fat, 66; nutritional content, 62; recipes with, 89, 90, 188–191
soy nuts, 46; nutritional content, 62
soy oil, 70; nutritional content, 62
Soy Pancakes, 176
soy powders, nutritional content, 64
soy proteins, properties of, 18–20
soy sauce, fragrant, 132, 134; light and dark, 48–49, 72
soy snacks, 60
soy sprouts, 17; nutritional content, 62
soy supplements, x
Soy-Banana Breakfast Drink, 89
Soybean Dip, 84
soybean oil, 17, 50–51
soybean sprouts, 49–50; nutrition content of, 166; recipe with, 163–166
Soybean Sprouts with Ground Pork, 163–164
Soybean Sprouts with Shredded Beef, 165
Soybean Sprouts with Shrimp, 166
soybeans, x, 17, 45; cooking dried, 76; nutritional content, 62; recipes with, 84, 105, 111, 144, 167
Spiced Roast Chicken, 138
Spicy Chickpeas, 120
Spicy Lentil Dip, 85
spinach, recipes with, 171–172
split peas, 17

Spring Rolls, 86–87
squash, 17
star anise, 137
Steamed Fish with Tofu, 153–154
Stewed Bean Curd Skin and Cloud Ears with Pork, 158–159
stir fries, 121–124, 147, 160, 168, 169
Stir-Fried Chinese Cabbage and Bean-Thread Noodles, 169
Stir-Fried Green Beans with Pine Nuts, 121–122
Stir-Fried Prawns, Snow Peas, and Tofu, 123–124
Stir-Fried Rice Noodles, 168
Stir-Fried Tempeh and Vegetables, 160
stock, 78; chicken, 77
Strawberry Soy Dessert, 188
Strawberry Soy Drink, 90
stroke, 3, 13, 33
sugar, 58
sulfur, 30–31
Summertime Pickled Curried Vegetables, 112–113
sunflower oil, 17
sunflower seeds, 17
surgery, 13
Sweet and Sour Tofu, 155
Sweet Potato Muffins, 183
sweet potatoes, 17, 24

Tacos (tofu), 143
tahini, 140; nutritional content of, 72
tamari, 72
tamarind, 73, 119
Tamoxifen, ix–x, 27
tea, 17; green, 38
tempeh, 51, 201; nutritional content, 62; recipe with, 160
Teriyaki Chicken, 139
texturized vegetable protein, 44, 51; nutritional content, 62
Thai Salad, 106
thrombin, 33
thrombosis, 13, 14

thyme, 3, 17
tofu, 47–48, 201; adding to diet, 61; nutrition content, 62; recipes with, 79, 80, 110, 123, 130, 143–159
tofu buk (deep-fried tofu), 73; recipe with, 87
Tofu Cutlet in Lettuce Leaves with Prawns, 161–162
tofu cutlets, 73; recipes, 80, 161–162
Tofu in Oyster Sauce, 148
Tofu Mayonnaise, 114
Tofu with Ground Meat, 151–152
Tom Yum sauce, 133, 135
Tomato Corn Chowder, 96
tomatoes, 24; recipes with, 96, 97
trans fatty acids, 29, 34
triglycerides, 32, 201
Tropical Fruit Smoothie, 91
tumors, 19
Tuna Soy-Mac Casserole, 174
turmeric, 3, 17
turnips, 30

uterine cancer, 14
uterus, ix

Vegetable Tofu Stir-Fry, 147
vegetables, 28; daily servings, 56; leafy green, 41
vitamin C, 36; sources of, 42, 50, 88, 125, 166
vitamin D, 41, 42, 45
vitamin E, 24, 36
vitamin K, 42

water, 58
water retention, 13
watercress, 30
weight gain, 13
West African recipe, 95
wheat, 17
wheat germ, 24

yams, 17
yogurt, 41

zinc, 47